With this body

With this body

CARING AND DISABILITY
IN MARRIAGE

Gillian Parker

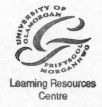

Learning Resources
Centre

Open University Press
Buckingham • *Philadelphia*

Open University Press
Celtic Court
22 Ballmoor
Buckingham
MK18 1XW

and
1900 Frost Road, Suite 101
Bristol, PA 19007, USA

First Published 1993

A catalogue record of this book is available from the
British Library

Library of Congress Cataloging-in-Publication Data

Parker, Gillian, 1952–
  With this body : caring and disability in marriage / Gillian
Parker.
     p.   cm.
  Includes index.
  ISBN 0–335–09947–5   ISBN 0–335–09946–7 (pbk.)
    1. Handicapped—United Kingdom—Marriage. 2. Handicapped—United
Kingdom—Family relationships. 3. Caregivers—United Kingdom.
4. Handicapped—Services for—United Kingdom.   I. Title.
HQ1036.P37   1992
306.87—dc20
                                                        92–18284
                                                        CIP

Typeset by Inforum, Rowlands Castle, Hants
Printed in Great Britain by Biddles Limited, Guildford and Kings Lynn

To Andrew·

Let me not to the marriage of true minds
Admit impediments. Love is not love
Which alters when it alteration finds,
Or bends with the remover to remove.
O, no! it is an ever-fixed mark,
That looks on tempests and is never shaken;
It is the star to every wand'ring bark,
Whose worth's unknown, although his height be taken.
(From Sonnet 116, William Shakespeare.)

Contents

Acknowledgements

The major debt of any researcher, is to those who provide the material on which this research is based. This book is no exception. My thanks go to the 22 couples who helped with the research by welcoming us into their homes and discussing their lives, and their hopes and fears for the future. I hope that giving them a voice through this book will go some way towards repaying their generosity.

As large a debt is owed to Maureen MacDonald, my co-interviewer. Without her skill and sensitivity as an interviewer, and the insight that she brought to bear on the topic of the research, the quality of the material used here would have been much poorer.

Thanks are also due to Audrey Cauwood of Relate (Marriage Guidance Council) who provided us with advice and support during the interviewing stage of the project, based on her wide range of knowledge and experience in the field of marriage and its problems. There is no doubt that her help made us better interviewers.

Sally Baldwin supervised the project on which the book is based with a light, but definite touch throughout and she, and other colleagues at SPRU, helped me to develop my ideas and thoughts into a coherent piece of research. Nikki Robus at OPCS selected the original sample of couples and made initial contact with them. Sara Graham at DHSS was the liaison officer involved in the project at its start, a post later taken over by Jenny Griffin and then by Madeleine Simms; Khalida Sheikh carried out the interviews in Urdu. Dorothy Thompson, Maggie Evans, Ian Robinson, Robert Anderson, Mr and Mrs Dodsworth, Mr and Mrs Craven, Mr and Mrs Buckle, and Mr and Mrs Ferguson all helped me to develop ideas before the research got under way. Robert Walker helped me give up my belief that truth could only be quantitative. Karl Atkin, Bryony Beresford, Anne Corden, and Julie Seymour have helped by commenting on various chapters of the book. Sue Medd and Jenny Bowes provided impeccable secretarial support throughout. My thanks go to all these people.

Another major debt is owed to those who took part in a series of seminars, funded by the Joseph Rowntree Foundation and held during 1991, which brought together disabled and non-disabled people, researchers and non-researchers, to discuss disability research. I believe that my thinking has developed and that this book has benefited as a result of the challenging discussions and exchanges which took place there. I doubt that any of the participants would agree with all that I have written here; but there would hardly be any point in writing the book if they did.

Finally, my thanks and love go to Andrew Cozens who provided emotional, intellectual and practical support throughout all stages of the research and the writing of the book, and whose bravery was, perhaps, the real inspiration behind it.

As always, any sins of omission or commission are mine alone.

This research was commissioned and funded by the Department of Health and Social Security (now Department of Health), but the opinions expressed are those of the author alone.

CHAPTER 1

The invisible marriage: disability and caring

Introduction

This book is about the experiences of married couples where one of the partners has become disabled or chronically ill since marriage. As such, it attempts to fill a number of important gaps in our knowledge of disability and caring.

First, research on informal care has tended to concentrate on those caring for older people (particularly when the carers are of a younger generation) or disabled children (see below). Yet, as recent evidence shows, carers of the *same* generation as those they care for, particularly spouses, make up a large proportion of those providing help and support to someone living in the same household (Green 1988). Spouse carers have never been the sole focus of British research in this field and younger spouses have been all but ignored.

Secondly, the experience of male carers has received little attention in the existing literature. By definition, many spouse carers are men; ignoring spouse carers has meant that male carers have also been effectively ignored.

Thirdly, despite the fact that there can be no informal caring without a disabled or frail older person to receive it, there have been few attempts to explore simultaneously and in depth the views and experiences of both 'actors'.

The personal origins of the study

The research on which the book is based had its genesis in a combination of personal experience and academic interest. In late 1983, while I was in the middle of carrying out a review of research on informal care, my husband developed a serious and potentially life-threatening illness. Having been immersed in accounts of the burden of providing care to relatives I was suddenly thrown into the position of imagining what my life and my husband's would be like if he were to become disabled, and I had to become his carer. I already knew from my literature review that we would be unlikely to get much in the way of supportive services or, at least, not ones that would enable me to continue working. In any case, would I or he really want anyone else to provide him with close personal care? If I gave up work to look after him what would my employment chances be after a protracted break?

We were extraordinarily fortunate in our experiences at that time. Acquaintances turned out to be friends, our colleagues at work were supportive, our employment circumstances allowed my husband to deal with his illness in his own time and allowed me to be with him when I wanted to, and, by and large, our families helped us to cope. Most fortunate of all, surgery and continued medical surveillance kept, and continue to keep, my husband well. However, the experience both changed us as individuals and changed our relationship, and still affects what we are and what we do. Furthermore, even beyond the obvious differences, both our short- and long-term reactions were different.

After the initial period of medical treatment was over my husband returned to work and I turned back to my review with a new and more personal interest. The first thing that I noticed was how very little of the available literature really addressed the position of younger disabled people and those who help them. My husband had not become disabled and had experienced something defined by all concerned as 'an illness'. However, had things not turned out so well (and at that early stage there was no guarantee about the outcome) we could have been faced with an indeterminate period during which he would have become increasingly ill *and* disabled. Neither the existing literature on caring nor that on disability had much to offer me in the way of insight about what that might be like.

I found myself puzzled by arguments that held that disability had nothing to do with illness or that belief in a need for some form of personal adaptation to impairment was essentially a form of false consciousness. I knew that disabled people argue that they should not be treated as if they were ill, but could see that many people who had impairments as a result of ongoing illness were also disabled. My unease increased as I watched my parents coming to terms with my mother's increasing impairments (and disability) related to arterial disease which left her tired and in almost continual pain. I could see that people can be disabled by their physical, economic and social environment but I could also see that people who become disabled (rather than being born with impairments) might have to renegotiate their sense of themselves both *with* themselves and with those closest to them. Also, looking around me, it seemed that many disabled people fall into categories where the argument that there should be no need for informal carers had less salience. How would couples who had been married for 20 years suddenly take to having paid assistance in the house for hours at a time if one of them became disabled? Might not disabled men who had been used to their wives providing them with domestic services and some forms of personal care insist on their wives being their main carers, even if sufficient resources were available for help to be bought in? Might not women like me, for all our allegiance to a feminist view of the world, *want* to provide at least some help and support to those whom we loved and might not they want the same from us?

I also found myself unhappy with some of the existing and developing literature on caring. The emphasis on those caring for disabled children and older people left some major question marks about how the feminist critique might apply to those looking after their partners. While I could appreciate (intellectually at least) that my feelings for my husband were constructed within a certain historical and political framework that was inherently oppressive for women, this did not alter the fact that they *were* feelings and that they were hurt when he was hurt. I was concerned, too, that we knew so little about what happens to relation-

ships when people become disabled and those close to them take on responsibility for help and support. Finally, in the absence of any statistics to support
the view that disabled women were any more likely to be divorced than disabled
men, it occurred to me that there must be at least as many younger men caring
for disabled wives as there were younger women caring for disabled husbands.
Men as carers were all but invisible in the existing literature and the developing
commentary on informal care implied that such male carers as there might be
had to be seen as aberrant. Yet I could not believe that, had our positions been
reversed, my husband would not have behaved and felt much as I did. What then
would the experience of men caring for wives be?

The aim of the review I had been writing when all this happened was to provide
an agenda for research on informal care for the British Department of Health and
Social Security (as it then was). I concluded that there was a need for research into
the informal care arrangements of younger physically disabled adults and suggested a study of married couples. This was funded in 1986 and completed in
1989.

The study

The small-scale, qualitative study of 21 younger (under pensionable age) couples,
where one partner has become disabled since marriage, which I then undertook
provides the empirical basis of this book. The couples were selected from a pre-
existing sample and were interviewed in their own homes, both together and
separately. More detail about how the study was carried out and some basic
information about the people who took part are given in the appendix. All the
names I have used are fictitious and some of the details of the people involved
have been changed to help preserve their anonymity.

The book illuminates two central issues that emerged from the study. The first
of these is that of dependence and independence, and how these are negotiated
both between the partners, and between the partners and the outside world of
family, friends, neighbours, employment, services and the physical environment.
The second is the way in which giving and receiving care are embedded within
pre-existing relationships. Those who acquire impairments in adulthood far out-
number those who are born with or grow up with impairments. Consequently,
the majority experience of disability and caring is within relationships which
may be well established.

The material in this book provides plenty of evidence for the social creation
model of disability which holds that disability is not 'an intrinsic feature of . . .
impairments but is created by a disabling and disablist society' (Oliver 1990: 85).
However, it also shows that the dynamics of pre-existing relationships, coupled
with age, gender and class, mediate the experience of disability and, therefore, of
caring.

The invisible marriage

Despite a burgeoning of research and comment on disability and on informal care
and carers, marriage has been strangely absent from discussion of either. Not only

has the relationship itself been missing, but so too has any recognition that, as things are currently, disability and caring are 'married' too. In an environment in which disabled people are largely prevented from meeting their needs for self-care other than through the agency of families and friends (see Chapter 4), it is inevitable that disability leads to informal care. This is not to argue that this is what *should* be but rather to acknowledge that this is what *is* and point to the need to look at the experiences of both participants. In the rest of this chapter I outline some of the reasons why I think that marriage, and the linking of disability and caring, have been ignored and what some of the consequences of this have been.

British research on 'informal care', so defined, really started with studies of families caring for severely disabled offspring, both children and adults (e.g. Bayley 1973; Wilkin 1979; Bradshaw 1980; Glendinning 1983, 1985; Baldwin 1985), but swiftly moved on to the provision of informal care to older people (e.g. Hunt 1978; Nissel and Bonnerjea 1982; Levin *et al.* 1983; Wright 1983; Wenger 1984; Ungerson 1987; Lewis and Meredith 1988; Qureshi and Walker 1989).

By contrast, there is no seam of studies about those who help and support younger disabled adults, particularly those who have physical impairments. Generally speaking, interest here has been confined to the psychological or medical literature, where issues of stress, coping and psychological adjustment are paramount (e.g. Kinsella and Duffy 1979; Korer and Fitzsimmons 1985; Livingston *et al.* 1985a,b; Orford 1987; Anderson and Bury 1988). There have been some accounts of people caring for younger, physically impaired people, but these have tended to be tucked away within books that have as their main focus the carers of older people or of children (e.g. Oliver 1983; Briggs and Oliver 1985; Hicks 1988). Information can also sometimes be gleaned from empirical studies of disabled people themselves (e.g. Sainsbury 1970; Blaxter 1976; Hyman 1977; Locker 1983). In 1985, a review of the British literature on informal care pointed to the scarcity of information about those who help and support younger physically impaired adults on an unpaid basis. A second edition of the review in 1990 came to the same conclusion (Parker 1985, 1990).

At the same time as the lives of those caring for disabled children and older people were being described, and sometimes in the same publications, a feminist critique of informal care was developing, pointing to the extent to which women were the principal care-givers, demonstrating the negative impact that this had on their employment, finances, and social and emotional lives and arguing for alternatives (e.g. Land 1978; Finch and Groves 1980, 1983; Baldwin and Glendinning 1983; Finch 1984; Dalley 1988).

To some degree the feminist critique was developed in reaction to an increasing emphasis in British social policy on 'care in the community' for disabled and older people. A series of policy documents during the 1960s, 1970s and 1980s promoted the move away from an emphasis on institutional or long-stay residential care towards community care for people who, for whatever reason, need help or support from others in their everyday living. The reasons for this shift in policy are complex. Research into the quality of accommodation and treatment in institutional settings (Townsend 1962; Goffman 1968; Morris 1969) and a series of public outcries about conditions in long-stay hospitals (Brown 1980) prompted change for certain groups of people, especially those with learning disabilities or mental health problems. The advent of psychotropic drugs which could control the symptoms of some psychiatric disorders also made care in community settings more achievable for people in the latter group.

At the same time, however, anxieties about the cost of providing institutional or residential care were also driving policy change. During the early 1960s British policy statements increasingly argued that the state was unable to bear the costs of expensive institutional care, and focused on the range and levels of statutory domiciliary and other services needed to sustain the continued independence of older or disabled people in the community. However, while the levels of community-based services did increase in response to these policy guidelines, the increases were rarely large enough to meet all the identified needs for these services (Walker 1982; Means 1986).

A further shift in emphasis took place in the mid-1970s, away from statutory provision of services towards the roles and responsibilities of family members as the primary providers of community care. Again finance was presented as a major driving force behind this shift. For example, the 1981 White Paper on services for older people, 'Growing Older' (Cmnd 8173) stated:

> Providing adequate support and care for elderly people in all their varying personal circumstances is a matter which concerns – and should involve – the whole community . . . Public authorities simply will not command the resources to deal with it alone. (para 1.11)

As a result, 'Care *in* the community must increasingly mean care *by* the community' (para 1.9, original emphasis). We will be exploring in more detail, in Chapter 4, a number of the implicit misunderstandings about the nature of care in the community contained in these statements. Their importance here lies in the assertion of the primacy of the informal provision of care for older people, a stance later carried over into policy documents concerning *all* disabled people (for example, Griffiths 1988; Department of Health 1989).

From the mid-1980s onwards a series of books and reports brought informal carers increasingly into the limelight; a process capped by their specific inclusion, for the first time ever, in British health and social services legislation (the Disabled Persons (Services, Representation and Consultation) Act 1986 and the National Health Service and Community Care Act 1990). This incorporation did not, however, raise questions about why so many disabled and older people had to rely on informal carers or posit alternative models of support for them. Rather, informal carers were seen as part of the natural background; a given source of support for disabled people (Twigg 1989).

The development of the feminist critique in Britain can be seen, therefore, as a response to these shifts in emphasis (Finch and Groves 1983). Demographic change, improvements in the medical care (and therefore, life expectancy) of children born with physical and mental impairments and of people seriously injured or ill in later life, and contracting family size, were all seen to increase the odds that any woman would, at some time, find herself responsible for the care of a disabled or frail family member. An increased emphasis on the provision of this care without the assistance of statutory services rang considerable alarm bells for many.

The developing critique, however, continued to concern itself with the care of children and older people and failed to deal with the issue of care for a partner.

Land and Rose (1985), for example, in outlining Ve's model of 'the altruistic basis of women's interactions with others' (p. 90), leap from 'care-giving work' for children and older people, to 'support between friends of approximately equal social power', via personal service between people 'who are both capable of self-care, but where the relations of power are unequal between them' (p. 90). As this latter is seen as characteristic of marriage and described by Land and Rose as 'compulsory altruism', partners providing help or support to younger disabled adults are totally invisible (as, indeed, are men, see below).

This absence continues even in the face of increasing evidence that the marriage relationship is the prime location of care, certainly for older people (Qureshi and Simons 1987; Ungerson 1987; Qureshi and Walker 1989). The only British study yet published which looks at both the givers and receivers of unpaid help and support, specifically excluded spouses by interviewing only helpers living outside the older person's own household (Qureshi and Walker 1989). Similarly, in her examination of the 'assistance and support which is exchanged within kin groups in adult life', Finch (1989) excludes 'specific discussion of responsibilities between spouses' because 'the responsibilities and duties associated with marriage specifically raise another set of issues which . . . are subject to regulation by law' (pp. 3 and 4).

This invisibility of marriage within the informal care debate has had a number of consequences.

Marriage makes it easier

First, commentators have made assumptions about disability and care within marriage that have no empirical basis and which, as we shall see throughout this book, are challengeable. One implicit assumption in some writing is that disability and caring within marriage will be in some way easier or at least less stressful than within other relationships. Borsay (1990), in reviewing other's writings, concludes that, despite any tensions that might arise if spouses have to reverse their accustomed roles:

> the management of disability in marriage is smoothed by ageing and the suspension of conventions pertaining to bodily care: retirement removes elderly males from the pressures of employment; older men and women may accept impairment and caring as an inevitable concomitant of old age . . . and fewer inhibitions ensnare cross-sex help between spouses with personal tasks like bathing and toileting . . . Care of elderly parents, and the role reversal entailed, is eased by no such moderating forces . . . (p. 114)

Apart from the implicit ageism of this analysis and that it ignores the fact that many disabled adults are both married and *young*, it also makes assumptions about 'cross-sex help' which, as we shall see in Chapter 2, are incorrect.

Mistaken assumptions about marriage are replicated in service provision, too, where the needs of younger disabled people are assumed to be met if they have non-disabled partners (Blaxter 1976; Morris 1989). This is a paradox because, as Dalley (1988) points out, one of the implicit reasons for the reliance on the 'reserve army' of (female) unpaid carers is the assumption that they 'are already provided for by being dependent on, and thus supported by, wage-earning men'

(p. 18). As we shall see in Chapter 5, many disabled men leave the labour market, while the lack of support for disabled women often affects their husbands' paid work. Neither male nor female partners of younger disabled people, then, are likely to be supported by anyone else's earnings.

Disabled women and male carers

Secondly, the lack of emphasis on marriage and the under-representation of women in accounts of disability has led to the virtual absence of men from any picture of informal caring. Studies of disabled children show that fathers rarely become involved to the same extent as mothers in the care of their children and when they do help out, it is often with the more pleasurable tasks (Wilkin 1979; Cooke 1982; Glendinning 1985). In this they are probably little different from other fathers. Similarly, when older people are being cared for in their married children's homes, men are far less involved in providing help and support, even when the parents are theirs rather than their wives' (Nissel and Bonnerjea 1982). However, when older or disabled people are living with a spouse the balance between male and female carers is, by definition, more even (Arber and Gilbert 1989).

Because the analysis of informal care has been driven so much by feminist scholarship, there has been a tendency to assume that any men who are heavily involved in caring are, in some way, aberrant. Dalley (1988) argues that, for men,

> the entanglement of caring for and caring about does not, broadly speaking, exist (and where it does, these men [*sic*] are usually regarded as atypical – in contrast to the case of women, where to *dis*entangle the processes is to be unnatural). Men, it is recognised, can care about, without being expected to care for. The conjunction for men, rather, is to care about and thus to *be responsible for*. Thus a man who refuses to take responsibility for chronically dependent members of his family is regarded as callous and beyond the pale, but he is not expected to provide the care (that is the tending) himself. (p. 12, original emphasis)

Dalley then goes on to develop her argument in terms of *sons* and *daughters*.

Even when spouses are specifically referred to, it is assumed that men would act differently from women. The men in Ungerson's (1987) study who were caring for wives were all retired. However, she states that even if this had not been the case, they would not have given up paid work in order to care. Rather they would have 'found someone else (the Social Services Department, a daughter, a paid employee or some combination of all three) to take it on, while they continued to earn enough to keep their wives and themselves in their accustomed environment' (p. 64).

This assertion begs many questions about the decisions these men might actually have made, but also fails to acknowledge the role of earnings, and thus of class, in men's ability to pay for substitute care (see Chapter 5). Furthermore, as will become clear from Chapters 3 and 4, neither other family members nor formal services are currently accessible to the majority of younger disabled adults and their partners as substitute sources of help.

Both sides of the coin

Disability and informal caring, in the absence of alternative models of support for disabled people, become different sides of the same coin; without the former, the latter would not exist. Some writers have acknowledged the shared disadvantage that disabled people and their carers experience (Dalley 1988; Jordan 1990; Morris 1991), but few have gone beyond this to explore how both individuals involved experience it. By and large, writers have stayed in their own camps. Feminists have tended to pose the needs of carers in ways that can be seen as in opposition to those of disabled people (see Morris 1991) while disabled people have asserted that they do not want care (and, therefore, do not include informal carers in their analysis, e.g. Wood 1991). There have been exceptions. Croft (1986), for example, has highlighted the dangers of current policies for community care 'increasing divisions and conflicts of interest between [carers and disabled people] instead of encouraging alliances and solidarity' (p. 34). Most recently, Morris (1991) has attempted to find a way across the divide by bringing the feminist perspective of disabled women to bear:

> Feminist research on carers is a valuable application of the principle 'the personal is the political' . . . However, the failure to include the subjective experience of 'the cared-for' has meant that the feminist analysis and strategies stemming from the research have a number of limitations. Most importantly it has resulted in a dilemma being posed between 'care in the community' *or* residential care, which is in many ways a false dichotomy. (p. 156, original emphasis)

Similarly, Graham (1991) points out that both community care policy makers and the feminists who criticize them have fused 'the location with the social relations of care'. Both have :

> yet to explore the conceptual distinction between . . . where care is carried out and the social relations that determine who gives and who gets care. The result is a mode of analysis which obscures forms of home-based care that are not based on marriage and kinship. (p. 65)

Furthermore, as I hope to show in this book, by looking at social relations within the home where caring takes place, a picture of both disability and caring emerges which is rather more complex than either the simple social creation model of disability or the feminist analysis of caring would suggest. This picture, I believe, presents a challenge to both these strands but also offers an opportunity for movement forward.

The language of caring and disability

I have tried, in writing the book, to follow the definitions of impairment and disability used by the disabled people's movement, that is:

> *Impairment* lacking part of or all of a limb, or having a defective limb, organism or mechanism of the body;
> *Disability* the disadvantage or restriction of activity caused by a contemporary social organisation which takes no or little account of people who have physical impairments and thus excludes them from the mainstream of social activities. (UPIAS 1976, cited by Oliver 1990: 11)

I have sometimes found it difficult to maintain the distinction, especially when describing the lives of people whose impairments arise directly out of an ongoing illness. All the disabled people in the study were, indeed, disabled according to the definition given above, but some of them were also dis-abled by their impairments, either intermittently or continuously, and often through pain and exhaustion, to such a degree that no change in social organization could significantly and permanently increase their participation in the 'mainstream of social activities'.

Generally speaking, I have used the words 'help and support' to describe what non-disabled partners did for their spouses. I have not, however, discarded the word 'carer' or, indeed, 'care'. Some disabled people argue that the assumption that they need care is oppressive and that talking about carers and care-receivers ignores or diminishes the extent to which they themselves give care, particularly in the case of disabled women (Morris 1991). I feel that it is too early to discard the words, particularly in a study that is about marriage where, for both women and men, caring about and caring for are inextricably linked, albeit that the ways in which they care *for* are different. I would also be unhappy about discarding a word that is closely bound up with so many women's self-image and one which has, to such great effect, made women's unpaid labour more visible.

In what follows, I usually refer to the disabled partner as 'the spouse' and the non-disabled partner as 'the carer'. I did not go into the research expecting to find that every non-disabled partner *was* the main provider of help and support. Indeed, I hoped I would find marriages where alternative sources of help had been established and suspected that, if I did, this would most likely be in cases where husbands were the non-disabled partners. In fact, although there were situations where spouses were getting some help and support from elsewhere, in no case did this come anywhere near the level of involvement of the other partner.

Limitations

Any piece of empirical research has its limitations; sometimes these arise from the methods used, sometimes from the topic itself and sometimes by chance. One of the limitations of the research that this book is based on is its inability to say much about the experience of disability and caring for black people. There was only one black couple in the eventual sample although it seemed that several others withdrew at the sample selection stage. The couple who were included were first language Urdu speakers and were interviewed by a first language Urdu speaker who was recruited specially. However, as explained in the appendix, the depth of the material obtained from these interviews was not the same as that for other interviews. The need for in-depth research on the experience of giving and receiving care among different ethnic groups is long overdue (Atkin and Rollings 1992).

Another limitation of the study was that the couples interviewed were almost all working class. The male spouses had mostly been involved in manual work, some of it very heavy, and were evenly split between those who were skilled and those who were semi-skilled. The female spouses and carers had almost all been in unskilled manual occupations. Although this bias limits to some degree the general applicability of the research, I feel that it could, in fact, help to redress the balance of some previous work on both disability and caring which has felt, to me at least, to have taken an uncritical, middle-class point of view. Despite the fact that so much disability is associated with manual occupations and with poverty, class has, until recently, been notable for its absence as a major analytical category in research on informal care and disability (Arber and Ginn 1991).

Finally, while this book is about marriage, disability and caring, it does not engage in a sustained way with the massive sociological or psychological literatures on marriage *qua* marriage. These literatures have, by and large, ignored disability in younger people in much the same way that the literatures on disability and caring have ignored marriage. The incorporation of either into the other is, I think, overdue but this book can only be a starting point.

Negotiating the boundaries:
physical and personal
care in marriage

In this chapter we explore the ways in which married couples in the study dealt with the personal and physical help provided to the disabled spouse. Before doing that there has to be some discussion about ideas and definitions of dependence, independence and interdependence. These ideas have been key to much of the debate in the disabled people's movement in recent years (Brisenden 1986; Oliver 1990) and I do not intend to go over this ground again. However, they need to be reviewed in order to understand fully some of the difficulties the couples in the study experienced. We also need to introduce a crucial distinction, which is not always fully articulated in the existing literature, between *expectations* about dependence and independence in self-care tasks, and the *achievement* of these tasks.

None of us, of course, is independent; we rely on each other in a multitude of ways from the provision of the essentials of food, water and shelter to the complexities of feelings of self-esteem. Furthermore, ideas about 'appropriate' levels of dependence or independence are not fixed, but vary with the nature of the tasks, the individual's age, gender, and physical and mental abilities, mediated through social, cultural, political and environmental forces, and across time. So, for example, no one expects babies to be independent in any sphere, but the age at which young children will be expected to become relatively independent economically, socially, emotionally or domestically will vary from society to society, from class to class, and between genders, and has varied across history. Normative notions of dependence and independence thus arise from a complex interplay of personal, social, economic, political and physical factors. In other words, ideas about dependence and independence are socially constructed.

At the same time, the extent to which individuals can or cannot achieve appropriate levels of dependence or independence is itself *determined* by these factors. For example, adults are generally expected to be able to get themselves from A to B with minimum intervention from others. Yet the degree to which they can is influenced by a physical environment largely designed for non-disabled people and an increasing emphasis on privatized forms of transport (the car) which exclude older and poorer people. Thus, dependence and independence are also socially created (Oliver 1990).

Dependence and independence in personal and physical self-care might, at first sight, seem to be least likely to be influenced by structural (economic, political, environmental) factors. The ability to feed and wash oneself, to get in and out of bed, to get up and down stairs, and to dress could be seen purely as a function of the individual's physical abilities and age. None of us can do these things when very young; most, but not all, acquire the requisite skills as we grow; some, but not all, will lose these as we age. A closer look, however, shows us that both expectations about, and the achievement of, these abilities are also influenced by the physical environment and, more subtly, by gender and economic factors. For example, there are probably few younger men who now expect to have their backs washed regularly by their wives or mothers. Yet, before the introduction of pit-head baths, whole communities of women expected and were expected to provide this form of personal care daily. Even when adults can feed and dress themselves a good proportion (mostly men) depend on someone else's having cooked the food and washed their clothes before they can do so. People with similar physical impairments may or may not be 'able' to feed and wash themselves, get in and out of bed, or up and down stairs, depending on whether or not their homes and the equipment in them are suitable. This, in turn, may be influenced by political decision-making about the level and quality of state help available to provide suitable housing or by the disabled person's own financial resources. This latter will, itself, be influenced by social and political attitudes towards disabled people in the labour market or towards levels of social security available to them. Thus, to say that a particular individual is 'unable' to perform some self-care task or 'needs' help with that task can beg a whole series of questions about the structures within and by which that inability or need is constructed and created.

Furthermore, disabled people have argued that definitions of dependence and independence based on what they are and are not able to do are inherently oppressive; independence is about control not about abilities:

> We do not use the term 'independent' to mean someone who can do everything for themself, but to indicate someone who has taken control of their life and is choosing how that life is led . . . The most important factor is not the amount of physical tasks a person can perform, but the amount of control they have over their everyday routine. The degree of disability does not determine the amount of independence achieved. (Brisenden 1986: 178)

Expectations that disabled people should learn to be as independent as possible, in the sense of being able to do things themselves, leads some to an exhausting and unremitting round of activities related to their personal and social care which leaves little energy for anything else (Sainsbury 1970). As a result, some have made a positive decision to be less 'independent' and to rely on formal or informal sources of help for personal and domestic care, in order to increase the scope for doing other things (Morris 1989).

Conventional notions of independence and dependence for women who have family responsibilities are even more complicated. Here, dependency is 'not absolute, but is conditional upon their being simultaneously depended upon by others. Thus, for many women, being a dependant is synonymous not with receiving care, but with giving it' (Graham 1983: 24). When disabled women are encouraged to be more independent then, it is often not so that they should be so for themselves, but in order that they should fulfil their assumed obligations to others:

> Aids and adaptations which are supposedly about helping us to be independent are in fact often about enabling others to be dependent on us for the tasks which keep a house clean and a family fed. Society's expectations of women being what they are, it is not surprising that many of us measure our 'success' or 'failure' in terms of whether we can return to the role of housewife and mother. (Morris 1989: 52)

We can think, then, about self-care on three different levels. First, there are normatively prescribed expectations about what different sorts of people (young and old; men and women; disabled and non-disabled) 'should' be able to do for themselves. Secondly, there are different ways of achieving self-care tasks oneself, influenced significantly by the economic and physical environment. Thirdly, there are ways of achieving independence through the agency of others, whether formally or informally.

As we shall see in the rest of this chapter, and throughout the book, all three levels were important for the disabled people in this study. Some felt acutely the challenges to expectations about what they should be able to do themselves and what their partners should have to do for them. Some found their physical and economic situation more favourable towards independence in self-care than others. However, all, in the absence of supportive services, found that they had to rely on the help of their partner to achieve independence in personal, physical and domestic self-care tasks.

Challenging expectations

The nature of help provided to disabled children and older adults by informal carers has been described in many publications (e.g. Bradshaw 1980; Glendinning 1983, 1985; Levin *et al.* 1983; Wenger 1984). The range of tasks identified in this study was not materially different from that found in these other studies: carers provided help with bathing, dressing, getting in and out of bed, and up and down stairs, toileting, medication and so on. What was different, of course, was the nature of the relationship between the carer and the disabled person – one which had previously been based on normative expectations about personal, physical and domestic care. While parents expect to provide care for their children, at least while they are infants, and adult children appreciate that they may, at some point, have to provide care for their parents, none of the people in this study had entered upon marriage expecting to need or to provide such help. The impact of this challenge to normal expectations about what a wife should or should not do for a husband, or a husband for a wife, ran through many of the accounts couples gave.

This is an important issue because as we saw in Chapter 1, there has been an assumption in the literature on informal care that care giving and receiving within marriage would, somehow, be *less* problematic than in other sorts of relationship (Ungerson 1983; Borsay 1990). As we shall see in what follows, this does not seem to be so.

Personal care

About half the carers helped regularly with bathing, washing and hair washing; another five helped intermittently or had done so regularly in the past. Spouses with the most seriously impaired mobility needed substantial help all the time – Mr Ord, for example :

> before he goes to bed at night he's got to be helped into the bath, you've got to lift him into the bath because, we sometimes find that if he has a bath it helps to relax his muscles. So you've got to lift him in, and then lift him out and dress him again.
> *Interviewer: How long does that take for you to give him a bath?*
> Oh, it must take three-quarters of an hour. Takes quite a while.

Other spouses were able to help themselves to some extent, but still needed the carer to be around when they bathed:

> I don't like him having a bath if I'm not in. So more often than not, when he's ready – he'll run the bath, he'll get in himself, but when he's ready for getting out, more often than not he will shout or knock, and then I'll go up and perhaps help him to rub his back, help him out, well he doesn't need a lot of helping, it's just a case of steadying him . . . (Mrs Clifton, carer)

Five spouses were helped with their toileting regularly and another five from time to time. In two cases, regular help included inserting catheters and/or changing catheter bags, and in one case manual evacuation of the spouse's bowels and help during menstruation. Mr Jefferson was the carer most heavily involved in regular intimate care. He evacuated his wife's bowels, changed her bladder catheter bags, and if the catheter came out or bypassed replaced it. He also had to help his wife while she was menstruating; both this and the manual bowel evacuation caused her acute distress:

> he has to put [sanitary pads] on [me] and I don't think that's right for a man . . . I mean I don't like it, he doesn't mind it but I hate it. I absolutely *hate* it and can't do nothing about it. (Mrs Jefferson, spouse)

This distress at being helped with intimate tasks was not confined to female spouses. Men were just as likely to feel uncomfortable with their wives helping them:

> if I can't get off the toilet, she has to help me that way. It's quite unpleasant some-times, it is for [wife].
> *Interviewer: Do you find this very hard to have to . . .*
> Hard? I find it hard and embarrassing . . . (Mr Gifford, spouse)

The provision of intimate care across sex boundaries has been argued by various researchers and writers in this field, most notably Ungerson (1983, 1987), to be problematic for carers. However, the problem has generally been characterized as one which is about the combination of *blood*-relationship and sex. By default, as we saw in Chapter 1, 'cross-sex caring' (Ungerson 1987) in relation to spouses has been assumed not to be problematic. Ungerson (1983) argued that:

> The fact that women have a virtual monopoly in dealing with these aspects of tending [dealing with incontinence and human excreta] can be most easily ascribed

to a system of taboo in contemporary British society about the management of human excreta. (p. 73)

Thus, she states, men are unlikely easily to become involved in tending incontinent people. Furthermore, because 'a great deal of tending necessarily and, in cases of incontinence, inevitably involves touching genitalia' (p. 74) then, when caring for kin, incest taboos will come into play. Consequently:

In the particular case of women carers looking after male relatives *other than their own husbands*, there is clearly a conflict between the demands of the taboos about human dirt which . . . effectively act to exclude men carers, and the taboos about incest. Hence such women may find themselves in exceptionally trying circumstances. (p. 75, my emphasis)

Evidence from this study, however, indicates that providing intimate personal care across sex boundaries does *not* become less problematic because the carer and disabled person are married.

Mr Jefferson, for example, felt that the personal care tasks which he carried out for his wife sometimes made it difficult for him to enjoy their sexual relationship. He expressed no distaste for what he did but he clearly found it difficult: '. . . when you've done all those sort of very personal things it takes the edge off it . . . it isn't as though the desire isn't there but it's like, as I said, . . . when do you stop being a nurse and become a husband'. Furthermore, as we saw earlier, Mrs Jefferson hated the fact that her husband had to provide intimate care.

Similarly, female carers had found it difficult to carry out certain tasks, especially initially, and their spouses had found it difficult to be helped in this way:

it's definitely harder looking after a man, looking after your husband because it's his feelings as well, you see, he doesn't *want* me to bath him but he can't do it himself and there's nobody else to do it . . . I don't mind, it's what I'm used to now but I wasn't used to anything like that and I didn't like the idea at first but it's what you've got to do . . . (Mrs Ibstock, carer)

Sooner or later, all these carers felt themselves to have got used to providing personal care for their spouses, usually because they had no choice but to do so. By contrast, some spouses, regardless of their sex, found it perennially difficult to come to terms with being cared for by their partners, both because of the nature of care that was required and because of the way in which it signalled unanticipated dependence:

[it was difficult to] think she had to help me like that . . . it still boils down to, you think how you were to what you are, and that's what makes you mad at the time, to think it could happen to you that way and that you're so dependent like a little baby, dependent on someone else. (Mr Ibstock, spouse)

Others said that, like the carers, they had got used to it, but that it had been difficult at first.

For several male spouses the embarrassment was clearly about the *sex* of the person providing the care because they had also found care from female nurses or doctors difficult to cope with, both initially and later:

when I first went in the hospital I was very embarrassed with the nurses, very, very –
until I got to know the nurses. They used to joke and smack me backside and all, have
a joke and a carry on, you know. Once you've got to know them they'd make you at
home. (Mr Keighley, spouse)

while he was in hospital he used to wait for me to come in and I'd end up doing it
and the bedpan and all that, he used to wait until I came in, the nurses all used to go
mad. (Mrs Mead, carer)

Mrs Jefferson used to wait for her regular visits to a Younger Disabled Person's
Unit to have an 'all-over' bath, because she so disliked her husband having to do
this for her. Mrs Newham, who was not at the stage of needing such intensive
help, also indicated that for women, as for men, the issue was about transgressing
sex boundaries:

it would worry me . . . I think I'd rather a woman than a man.
Interviewer: Would you?
Yes, I think I would, yeah. I'm still a bit naive – not naive, a bit private. I suppose I've
always been like that . . . I wouldn't like [husband] to have to put my pants on and
things like that, I think I'd be a bit embarrassed, I don't know why, shouldn't do
really, should I?

Mrs Newham's puzzlement about *why* she should find the prospect of receiving
personal care from her husband, when she shared a bed and a sexual relationship
with him, perhaps goes some way to explaining why other commentators have
assumed that caring for a spouse would be less problematic than cross-sex caring
for a blood relative. What we have found here is that being married does not
magically dispose of the embarrassment we are brought up to feel about our
bodies and nudity, or of the psychological difficulties that come when we feel
that we are challenging 'normal' boundaries. Rather, having a marital partner
provide personal care can be *more* difficult because it may also interfere with the
couple's sexual relationship (see Chapter 6).

By examining the views of both the disabled person and the carer it has been
possible to show that difficulties associated with personal care are not limited to
the carer. Both partners found it difficult and the spouse's feelings could compound difficulties for the carer. Most people became inured to the situation – in
the absence of supportive services it had to be; therefore, they bore it – but this
made it no easier.

Some spouses' reluctance about being cared for by professionals, which we will
explore further in Chapter 4, raises obvious difficulties in regard to thinking
about how disabled people and carers should be supported. However, this was not
a homogeneous group. One of the most seriously disabled spouses, Mr Ord, did
say that he found professional care easier (albeit that he had refused when offered
it, see Chapter 4):

If you are being cared for by a nurse, in a hospital, it's not embarrassing, everyone
else is in, more or less, the same position as you . . . But I can remember for ages and
ages . . . if I wanted to move my bowels I couldn't even wipe my own bottom. Now to
ask your wife to do it is embarrassing, for some reason or another, to ask a nurse to do
it wasn't embarrassing. In fact they'd joke and they'd laugh about it, they were
trained to do it.

Mr Ord's comments show that not all people feel the same way about being cared for by professionals, even if they cross sex boundaries, and that the provision of services to carry out intimate care, when appropriate, would support carer and disabled person alike. When the disabled person does not want professional care of this sort, and when the carer can cope with providing this sort of care, then service providers need to find some other form of helping input.

Physical care

As well as the personal help which carers provided, they also helped with physical tasks – helping their spouse to get in and out of bed, and up and down stairs, and with dressing and feeding.

Almost half the spouses needed regular help getting in and out of bed, and another two had to be helped from time to time. Even those spouses who were relatively mobile once upright were likely to need help of this sort, particularly when they had chronic back problems. Some carers and spouses developed quite complex routines to deal with the difficulty:

> [when he gets back into bed] he sort of gets hold of my foot and I'm prising him down, down the bed you see using my foot as a lever. It's funny but it works. He'll say, 'Give me your foot' and I'll bring me knee up like that and he'll get hold of me feet and then I'm pushing him, like levering him down until he gets far enough down and then I hold, put my hand on side of his neck there to take [the weight] so that his arm can, you know, to let him flop back like that. (Mrs Clifton, carer)

The need for help getting in and out of bed was, obviously, closely associated with the need for help in the night and several carers gave help or attended to their spouses regularly or occasionally in the night. Others had their sleep disturbed most nights by their spouses' restlessness in bed or getting up in the night: 'Sometimes he's so restless you know – he gets cramp and he has to get out of bed and walk the floor. And I'm rubbing the muscles of his legs, to try and relax them a bit . . .' (Mrs Baker, carer).

Those caring for the most disabled spouses were the ones most regularly disturbed at night: 'if he's really sore I've been woken up with him screaming with the pains in his legs, some nights you're up every hour'. (Mrs Ord, carer).

Spouses sometimes tried to avoid disturbing their partners in the night and tried to cope by themselves, but this could make things worse:

> She has to get me up in the night – sometimes I try to get up meself and I fall and she hears the bang and then she's upset and gets on to me. She's annoyed at me for not waking her but, I mean, it's worse because then she's got a job to get me up again to go to the toilet. (Mr Keighley, spouse)

The extent of regular help with dressing varied from help putting on shoes and socks for those spouses who could not bend to the complete dressing of Mrs Jefferson and Mr Selsdon:

> having to get [wife] dressed is not an easy job. Her legs are bent double underneath her and if I've got to try to do it without actually hurting her, I can't rush into it, I've got to gradually move her over, pull one side of her skirt or trousers or whatever . . . (Mr Jefferson, carer)

A few spouses also needed regular help getting up and down stairs. As with getting in and out of bed, several couples had developed special 'routines' to help them cope:

> we just work it out [when his back gives way], she'll just say to me, 'All right, just lay there a minute, and we'll sort something out' . . . and we get round it. We always have done. (Mr Gifford, spouse)

Only one spouse needed help with eating regularly, but others had either needed help in the past or needed help intermittently. This sort of help was a new development for Mr and Mrs Ord, and seemed likely soon to become a regular feature of their lives: 'if his hands have got a tremble you sometimes have to feed him, which has just lately come on, he gets this terrible tremble in his hand and he can't quite get the fork to his mouth'.

Some carers regularly provided help with or took total responsibility for their spouses' medication. Sometimes this took the form of watching for symptoms and encouraging the spouse to take the appropriate medication:

> There's not much you can do really [when husband has a fit], you just make sure he can't hurt himself. I mean, he takes tablets every day for the fits and if I sort of see he's going off I try to get a couple of tablets into him straight away. (Mrs Selsdon, carer)

In other cases it was a matter of seeing that the right tablets were taken at the right time.

One carer was actually responsible for dressing her husband's wound in the evenings and played the role of 'dirty nurse' in the mornings when the district nurse visited:

> [while getting breakfast ready] I'm rinsing his dish out for when the nurse comes, getting his pot out for his distilled water, I have to heat that up. Then get trays ready for nurse when she comes . . .
>
> I help the nurse when she comes, I'm what they call the dirty nurse. I tear all the packets, it's all got to be sterile, so up 'till this last three weeks about I have been dressing his wound myself at night for the last three . . . yeah, three years more or less, I have dressed it at night. I don't irrigate the wound, but I clean it all and do that. But at the moment it's dry, there's no infection. (Mrs Derby, carer)

Watchfulness: negotiating dependence and independence

As well as the practical tasks they carried out for their spouses, carers also mentioned the watching out that they undertook. This ranged from making sure that other members of the household did not leave things on the floor for the spouse to trip over, through being around in case anything went wrong, to quite complex medical decision-making about the spouse's state of health and the need for intervention. It could also involve protecting the spouse from doing too much.

Some couples had particular difficulties negotiating an appropriate level of watchfulness. Spouses, in their desire to maintain their independence, could sometimes make life more difficult for their partners. We have already seen that Mr Keighley's attempts to get himself to the toilet during the night could be counter-productive. The degree of 'watchfulness' the carers had developed was related to the nature of the spouse's impairments, to the length of time since they had started and to the carer's other responsibilities. The carers of people with chronic back or joint problems, which really *could* be triggered off by doing too much or twisting awkwardly, were usually the most anxious but, in some cases they had come to an accommodation over time:

> I think I've evened myself out when it comes to [helping husband]. See, after ten years you do get – at one time you want to do too much but like I said, you've got to give him so much leeway. He's got to be independent himself 'cos like I say, if I'm ever ill he's got to be able to cope with him hisself, you see. (Mrs Gifford, carer)

When spouses had been gravely ill or suffered from life-threatening conditions, the temptation for carers to be *too* watchful once the crisis had passed was great. Mr Derby had been extremely ill and had not really been expected to live. More than five years of devoted care from Mrs Derby and several hospitalizations had brought him to the point where he was much better, had started to gain weight and to move around again. Mr Derby's wish to regain some degree of independence, although a great joy to Mrs Derby as a sign of his improving health, also triggered anxiety:

> *Interviewer: Do you ever do more for him than is strictly necessary?*
> No, he wouldn't let me.
> *Interviewer: Have you tried?*
> Yes – do you want [his] answer, even though it is on tape?
> *Interviewer: If I may.*
> 'I'm not a bloody invalid.' So, you know, I only have to do what is needed because no way would he put on me if that's what you mean . . .
> *Interviewer: And have you felt the need yourself to do things for him, to protect him?*
> Yes, I have, and this is when I get that answer, you see, if he's going to do anything new that he's not done before then I'm always wary that it's going to upset him and we're going to be back where we started, so I obviously – yeah, I do mother him a bit I suppose.
> *Interviewer: But he sets limits to that by . . .*
> Yes, definitely.
> *Interviewer: . . . by telling you where to stop?*
> That's right. I think we've got a pretty good balance there because I can natter on and natter on and he'll do what he wants anyway if he can, because I'll say, 'I shouldn't risk that, do you think you ought to?', but if he thinks he can he will and he's a trier and once it's done then I'm all right, I know it's not hurt him and another barrier we've got over. (Mrs Derby, carer)

For this couple, and for others, it had been possible to negotiate an appropriate level of 'watchfulness', but the process of doing so had not been without costs for the carer. Other couples had not negotiated this process successfully with the result that spouses interpreted their wife's or husband's watchfulness as interference or fussiness.

There were real conflicts of interest here for some couples; while both partners might want to help to maintain the independence of the disabled spouse, at the same time carers wanted to protect their spouses against doing too much and harming themselves. This was, of course, because they did not want to see them in pain, but also because they knew that it would be they – the carers – who would 'pick up the tab':

> *Interviewer: You don't sometimes do a bit more for him because you can do it faster or . . . ?*
> Well, I *can* do it faster but it, it's an effort for him, so why give him the effort when I can do it for him, you know. I mean it's no good him just sort of getting himself all antagonised over one little job what I can do for him. (Mrs Baker, carer)

> *Interviewer: Do you ever do more for [wife] than is strictly necessary?*
> I don't think it's more than necessary. I think it is *necessary*, you know what I mean, 'cos, I'll tell you something, sometimes, over the years, she'll attempt to do things and then as soon as she gets going she's got to knock off again. And I'll say, 'Go and sit down' 'cos she just can't cope. (Mr Eden, carer)

By contrast, there was another group of carers who felt that, if they allowed it, their spouses would become too dependent on them or, in some cases, had actually done so. Some resisted this process, feeling that it was better for the spouse to be kept independent, others resented it because of the demands it made on them, and others just put up with it:

> I mean it's so easy if he's doing anything for him to say, 'Would you mind passing me that there' and without thinking, you find out you're passing it. But if I think, I say, 'No, you're quite capable of going and getting that yourself', [and he says] 'Well, I suppose I am' . . . you know, it's just habit, 'Will you pass me that?' and if I can think I'll say, 'No, go and get it' (laughs). (Mrs Clifford, carer)

> Sometimes, just because I'm there, can be rather – how can I put it? – instead of really doing something for herself she'd say, 'Oh, [husband]'ll do it' – and it causes quite a lot of problems because I'll say, 'No, you do it', and she'll say, 'No, I'm not going to do it, that's what you are here for'. (Mr Jefferson, carer)

Although 'watchfulness' is, by definition, not as visible a task as are those connected with everyday living activities, this section has shown how important it was. Carers spent time protecting their spouses 'from themselves' and sometimes from others. By doing so they hoped to preserve the spouse's health and prolong his or her independence. Paradoxically, however, this protection was sometimes seen by spouses as lessening their independence. By contrast, other carers spent time encouraging their spouses to be more independent, risking being considered tough or heartless in the process (cf. Locker 1983: 149). For the most part the boundaries between dependence and independence were negotiated between the partners; occasionally either carer or spouse had just given in, allowing the other partner to determine the boundaries alone. The conflict that arose in such situations could be harmful to the partners' relationship – a problem which is examined further in Chapter 6.

Conclusion

This chapter has shown that the nature and range of caring activities carried out by wives and husbands for their disabled spouses are very like those identified in studies of other groups of carers and disabled people. We have also seen that giving and receiving personal care between married couples is no less problematic than it is in other relationships. Indeed, it may be the case, for some married couples at least, that it is *more* problematic. The low level of provision of services to younger married couples (see Chapter 4) and their relatively unsupported position in informal networks (Chapter 3), coupled with the need to provide or receive substantial help, and psychological resistance against doing so, may create great stress for both partners and seriously undermine the marital relationship. These issues will be discussed further in Chapters 6 and 8.

This chapter has also posed some difficult questions about how disabled people and their carers can best be helped and supported. There has been a tendency in the writings of the disabled people's movement to assume that redirected and/or increased resources which would give people the freedom to arrange their own lives would solve the dependence/independence issue: '[this notion of independence] can be applied to the most severely disabled person who lives in the community and organises all the help or "care" they need as part of a freely chosen lifestyle' (Brisenden 1986: 178).

One can see that this ideal can work for single adults. It can also work for adults who marry after they have established their independent lifestyle as long as they and their partners negotiate their feelings about the presence of a third party in the relationship. It is more difficult to see how it would work within established marriages when one partner becomes disabled. Some spouses found receiving personal care from their partners difficult; but others, particularly men, found the idea of care from an outsider even more so. As we will see in later chapters, some spouses had turned down offers of professional help with personal and physical care while some carers had themselves refused help, knowing that their partner would find it unacceptable.

In the absence of other helpers, does the partner become part of the help and care that the disabled person organizes him or herself? How do pre-existing patterns of power within the marriage influence the disabled partner's ability to choose freely or, indeed, the carers' ability to refuse freely. These are crucially important questions which existing literature on disability (with its emphasis on younger, often single, men) and on caring (with its emphasis on carers of older people) has all but ignored.

C H A P T E R 3

'They've got their own lives to lead': the role of informal networks

Introduction

In the previous chapter we explored some important issues around the giving and receiving of personal and physical care in marriage. In this chapter, we expand our view to take in the potential role of helping networks beyond the married couple: their children, other relatives, neighbours and friends.

There has been a strong emphasis in recent policy on the provision of help to disabled and frail older people through informal and voluntary networks. The 1981 White Paper 'Growing Older', in a now much-quoted phrase, asserted that:

> the primary sources of support and care for elderly people are informal and volun-
> tary. These spring from the personal ties of kinship, friendship and neighbourhood
> . . . It is the role of public authorities to sustain and, where necessary develop – but
> never to displace – such support and care. Care *in* the community must increasingly
> mean care *by* the community. (DHSS 1981: para. 1.9, original emphasis)

More recently, and more generally, Sir Roy Griffiths' 'Agenda for Action' on community care stated that families, friends, neighbours and other local people would 'continue to be the primary means by which people are enabled to live normal lives in community settings' (Griffiths 1988: para 3.2).

The impetus to promote care in the community as an ideal has, until recently, been based on the assumption that living outside large-scale institutions, and preferably with family members, is in the best interests of disabled and older people, and is in accordance with their wishes, and those of their families and friends. The aims of policy have been, on the one hand, to promote independent living among people in long-stay residential settings to enable them to move into the 'community' and, on the other hand, to promote independent living among those currently in the community who might be at risk of entering residential care.

However, other political issues have also promoted an emphasis on care in the community. Since the mid-1970s official policy statements have increasingly argued not only that the state cannot bear the costs of institutional care, but also that it cannot afford to provide a comprehensive network of health and welfare services to support the many older or disabled people who live in the community. Again the White Paper 'Growing Older' articulated this view clearly:

> Providing adequate support and care for elderly people in all their varying personal circumstances is a matter which concerns – and should involve – the whole community . . . *Public authorities simply will not command the resources to deal with it alone.* (para 1.11, my emphasis) *So does that mean ends, are community has to deal with it alone?*

This combination of financial considerations with the avowed aims of promoting care in the community has led to an inevitable shift in emphasis from statutory provision (which is seen as expensive) to informal and voluntary provision (which is seen as inexpensive or even free) as a means of implementing policy. The 'first task of publicly provided services' has thus become 'to support and where possible strengthen' informal networks (Griffiths 1988: para 3.2).

The new role for the state, then, is not to encourage self-directed independence for disabled and older people, but rather to maintain dependence on family and other informal networks or, in some cases, effect a transfer of dependence from the state to the family/neighbourhood. The logical outcome is not reduced dependence for the individual, but rather the promotion of reliance on informal networks as intrinsically good or better than reliance on formal sources of help. Thinking in terms of the three levels of independence outlined in Chapter 2, independence of a sort is achieved, but only at the expense of increased dependence on others who are not paid for their work. Carer and cared-for person are, thus, locked into a relationship that neither may wish for.

Furthermore, the promotion of informal and voluntary provision is based on a number of inaccurate propositions. One of these is that 'the community' (rarely defined) does not do as much as it could do to help disabled or older people. As a result, there is a related proposition that a large, untapped and dormant reserve of help exists within kinship, neighbourhood and friendship networks. This, it is implied, if only given the right sort of encouragement would spring into life thus reducing or even doing away with the need for state-provided services. A further proposition is that reliance on informal sources of help is what disabled or older people themselves want.

How well do these propositions stand up against the evidence?

First, there is little evidence to suggest that the community does not care. The proportion of older people who live in the community rather than institutional or residential care has changed little since the turn of the century (Parker 1990). Even given recent developments in the provision of private residential care in the United Kingdom, the vast majority of disabled people still live in the community, regardless of the nature of their disability (Martin *et al.* 1978). Secondly, the incidence of informal caring activity is high. The 1985 General Household Survey (GHS) showed that one adult in seven in Great Britain was providing some service to a disabled or older person and that one in five households contained an informal helper (Green 1988).

Secondly, while informal help may be substantial, to talk about informal 'networks' in relation to community care is misleading because the involvement of neighbours and friends overall is not great. The GHS report showed that 13 per cent of adults were helping a relative but only four per cent a friend or neighbour (with some overlap between the two). In other words, informal 'networks' are predominantly family 'networks'. Furthermore, shared responsibility between family members, even in the same household, is relatively unusual. Once one person has been identified as a carer, other relatives, friends or neighbours rarely contribute (Parker 1990).

Thirdly, if we turn to the personal and intimate care with which disabled and older people often need assistance, family help becomes even more predominant. Neighbours, friends and less close kin rarely provide help with such tasks (Bulmer 1987; Qureshi and Simons 1987; Parker 1990).

Finally, while disabled and older people want to live in their own homes with their families or friends, this does not mean that they necessarily want their families and friends to provide them with extensive help or support. As long ago as 1963 Rosenmayr and Kockeis used the phrase 'intimacy at a distance' to describe older people's ideal relationship with their families. As we saw in Chapter 2, the same can be true of younger disabled people in relation, particularly, to their personal care, even within marital relationships.

Recent innovations in service management and delivery which attempt to develop informal help and then to mesh it with that provided from the statutory sector have failed to recognize any potential problem in the involvement of informal carers (Davies and Challis 1986). Nor have they recognized that continued or increased reliance on informal help might have costs for both receiver and giver beyond those measured in experimental schemes (Dant and Gearing 1990; Parker 1991). As Morris has pointed out, disabled people 'have complicated feelings about receiving help; on the one hand helpers can bring about independence, on the other their very necessity can make us feel helpless and dependent' (Morris 1989: 42).

In summary, while the community (or at least families) *do* care, serious questions have to be raised about whether this reliance is right. Furthermore, evidence presented in the rest of this chapter, calls into serious question whether informal help from beyond the immediate family *could* be activated and, if it could, whether it would be acceptable to disabled spouses and their partners.

We will look, in turn, at issues around help from children, other relatives, neighbours and friends.

Help from children

All but one couple had children and fourteen still had offspring living with them, but few received substantial practical help or support from this source. Furthermore, when help was given it was more likely to be with domestic tasks or household maintenance than with personal or physical care. On the few occasions when children had helped to look after their disabled parent it had been because the carer was physically incapable of doing so, usually because of their own illness.

Some adult children provided transport for the couple; a very important form of help for those who were unable to drive or could not afford to run a car (see Chapter 5). Others helped by providing either direct financial support or help in kind which eased the parents' budget. This was often a feature of help-giving where children did not have the time to give practical help or were too far away to do so. For example, Mrs Baker said several times throughout her interview that she could not expect her family to help out because they lived away, were working, had family responsibilities of their own or all three. However, the family did provide sensible presents of clothing or shoes, for Christmas or birthdays, and occasionally made contributions to the domestic economy:

> me eldest daughter, she came up. She brought me that big box of soap powder and a big Comfort. Now that's a great help for me, for washing. Them's sensible presents . . . well, it wasn't a present, it was . . . well, a gift. You know what I mean? A gift. Yeah, she says, 'Mother, you'll need it'. 'Cos she's a bit, she works herself like and she's pretty good like that, you know. And anything that's going. (Mrs Baker, carer)

In some cases financial help was in the form of treats or outings, or towards leisure equipment to help compensate for the couple's restricted social life:

> they helped out with things in kind, you know . . . We bought that video because it was on offer. Because we don't go to the cinema, we don't go to the theatre, and for what it costs, well we paid cash for it, but daughter helped us . . . (Mr Derby, spouse)

Out of context, the level of provision of help from children seemed low. However, it was clear that particular sets of conditions had to be met before offspring *could* help.

Proximity

As other work on informal care has indicated (Qureshi and Simons 1987; Glendinning 1988) the most important, and most obvious, factor enabling children to help is their presence in the home. Mrs Clifton described how her adult son helped his father with bathing and other tasks while he was still living at home. For Mr Linton, the presence of adolescent children in the home meant that he no longer had to take days off work after his wife had an epileptic fit. The return of Mr and Mrs Eden's son, after the break-up of his marriage, had been a blessing in disguise, especially when the carer, Mr Eden, became ill himself: 'we've been lucky in that respect. I mean I know it's terrible to say that his marriage broke up but we helped him through that patch and he's been able to help us through this' (Mrs Eden, spouse).

Yet, when asked if she would have looked to her son for help had he been living away from home Mrs Eden was adamant that she would not. The fact that he was at home meant that she did not have to *ask* and it was asking that was problematic. Thus, actually being in the home could remove or reduce one of the barriers to help from children.

Just as being there was the most important factor in determining help from resident children, so being near was an important factor with non-resident children: 'They'd be there within minutes if I need it – well the two local ones would, I mean me daughter that lives at C., it's not quite as handy for her to get over' (Mrs Clifton, carer).

For those children who were not in the immediate vicinity, access to a car was important: 'I can rely on them providing that they've got their cars on the road' (Mrs Derby, carer).

Having resources

We have seen that some children helped their parents financially or with help in
kind which relieved the parents' household budget and that this help sometimes
appeared to be given in lieu of practical help. Obviously, only those offspring
who were themselves prosperous or at least had some excess of income over needs
were able to help in this way. Thus, Mr and Mrs Derby did not expect their son to
run about in his car on their behalf when he was unemployed, but were very
grateful when his unemployment meant that he could help out with garden and
household maintenance.

Mr and Mrs Baker's children were all away from home, some at a distance, but
all had fairly well paid jobs and helped out whenever they could: 'they'll ring me
up. "Does me dad want anything?" Anything like that, anything in particular'
(Mrs Baker, carer).

Even where offspring were not particularly prosperous, just the fact of having a
job could help parents out, especially where the child was still resident. By contrast, unemployed offspring, even when no longer resident, could be a financial
drain on their parents.

Children with excess resources, then, tended to help out financially or in kind,
but the existence of an excess was, inevitably, determined by their own paid
work. However, paid work, particularly when away from their home town for
sons, and particularly when full-time or combined with child-rearing for daughters and daughters-in-law, reduced the amount of practical help they could give.
The availability of financial resources was thus, at one and the same time, the
reason why children could not help out practically *and* an alternative to practical
help. By contrast, when children were without paid work and other responsibilities, and were at home or nearby, their practical help could be an alternative
to financial help.

As we will see in Chapter 5, money, or the lack of it, was a pressing issue for
many of the couples included in the study. Access to financial or quasi-financial
resources via their children could, therefore, be very important.

'They have their own lives to lead'

Even when children lived at or near to home they did not always help out or help
to any great extent. In many cases respondents explained this in terms of the
children having their own lives to lead. This was an extremely important constraint from the parents' point of view – making many of them reluctant to ask
for help and even more reluctant to accept proffered help. There were several
elements to the children having their own lives to lead.

First, there were those who had their own families to care for:

> They're very good if I need them – very, very good if I need them. But like I say, they've
> got families of their own, they've got their own lives to lead and I don't put them under
> no obligation to do anything, but if I need help they're there. (Mrs Baker, carer)

Secondly, parents did not expect great amounts of help when their children or
partners – particularly daughters or daughters-in-law – had paid work. By contrast, as we have already seen, unemployment might provide opportunities for
giving practical help:

well I don't do much to help her, you see. I've a son that's on supplementary benefit at the moment, what happens after he starts work, well we don't know.
Interviewer: He helps out a lot does he?
Oh yes, he helps with the garden, you know. He does the hoovering and the cleaning of the hearth . . . and if the wife does blankets and all that he takes them out and hangs them on the line . . . (Mr Fowey, spouse)

Thirdly, there were the children who had their own problems – who were unemployed or divorced or single parents or, in one case, had health problems in their own family.

Attitudinal barriers

There was a second, related, constellation of constraints regarding help from children which was less about the objective, external demands of jobs and families, and more about the subjective, internal barriers of the parents' own attitudes. These constraints applied as much to resident as to non-resident children. The first element here was to do with parents not *expecting* their children to help out, sometimes explained as due to the carer's belief that it was her or his duty to care:

say I want him [son] to look after my wife while I do something else, he'd have to do it . . . but regarding anything [else], I don't think I'd bother really . . .

'cos I don't know what it is, whether it's being pig-headed or what, I don't know really. I feel it's me duty while his mother's not well and I feel it's me duty to do it, you see, and that's it. (Mr Eden, carer)

The second element, particularly for carers, was the constraint about not wanting to use up help from children, but to keep it in reserve for when it was really needed:

I prefer to [manage], because I don't know how long I'm going to be able to manage on me own – you see I may need their help sometimes so I don't want to be always on at them to come and do me this and come and do me that. (Mrs Clifton, carer)

This attitude was evident also in Mrs Derby's insistence on paying her daughter-in-law for her help with heavy housework.

Thirdly, there was a complex set of constraints which were about protecting people: protecting children from full knowledge about their father's or mother's impairments, and protecting spouses from the assumed shame that would come from the children's knowing:

I daresay all I've got to do is go down and knock on the door or pick the phone up and say, 'Would you come up', 'cos I mean our [son]'s said time and time again, 'Mam, if you want any help you've only got to phone', but I don't want the two of them to see their dad like that when he's at that stage where he can't help himself. (Mrs Ibstock, carer)

Age, gender and the nature of help provided

There was a further set of constraining factors, some of which overlapped and interacted with each other and with those already identified, which concerned age, gender and the type of help which might be provided.

First, it was obvious that where there were dependent children, or children who had been dependent at the onset of the parent's disability, help giving was not as frequent. This was usually explained by parents as being due to the children's age:

> She may be able to help me more as she gets older . . . she's probably more aware of things but you see, you can't put, I don't like to put too old a head on her, not at nine year old – they've got to go through their childhood, and they should go through it properly – so I don't like to overload her mind with things that she shouldn't be bothered with at the moment. (Mr Gifford, spouse)

Sometimes the consideration of age was also tied in with the appropriateness of asking a child to carry out particular types of task, especially those related to personal care. Sometimes this was coupled with anxieties about gender:

> It's difficult because . . . me daughter, she's only nine. She understands a lot of me problems and she does help in some ways but you really mean personal [care] – deep down, personal, which you can't involve your own daughter at that age. (Mr Gifford, spouse)

However, it could just as well be about the personalities of the children involved:

> it's not fair to ask lads, sons, to come and deal with her when she's had one of the 'dos' [fits] because she's got to be changed, undressed and bathed, like.
> *Interviewer: So is it your daughters you mostly call on for help?*
> The eldest, not the youngest, the youngest couldn't cope with it. (Mr Linton, carer)

However, regardless of their age boys were often seen as unlikely sources of help.

Age, gender and the nature of the tasks were thus seen by parents as constraints to their children helping out. However, the gender constraint and, in at least one household, the age constraint were overcome when there was no alternative. Thus, Mrs Clifton's son helped with caring for his father because, when severely ill, he was too difficult for Mrs Clifton to manage on her own; Mrs Eden's son cut her toe nails for her because Mr Eden's eyesight was not up to the task; and both he and Mr and Mrs Quincy's young daughter took on considerable responsibilities when *both* their parents were ill.

Help from other family members

Kinship networks

Only one couple had any kind of kinship network capable of or willing to deliver help on a regular basis. Fewer than a third of carers and fewer than a fifth of spouses had both their parents alive, while a third of carers and over half the spouses had neither parent alive. Over a half of both carers and spouses had living siblings but few saw them regularly and fewer still received any help from them. In all, only a half of the couples mentioned any form of help or support from their extended family.

The help received was mostly with transport and household maintenance rather than domestic tasks or helping the disabled spouse. Indeed, in only two cases had there been any substantial input from relatives with personal or domestic tasks and in both cases this had been from the disabled spouses' parents:

> there was one time I was really rough and my mother and father came 'cos . . . I don't know how [wife] managed 'cos I wasn't always as thin as this . . .
>
> It was before they took us into hospital in 1983, I couldn't get out of bed, I was hopeless, and she used to have to help us out of bed into the bath and . . . have to lift us into the bath, you know, to bath us, it was all right getting us in but getting us out, I was slippy . . . but me dad came this time to help us in and out the bath, a couple of times, that's about all. (Mr Ibstock, spouse)

Mr Ibstock's parents had also looked after him while his wife had been in hospital.

That this sort of help came only from the parents of the disabled spouse seems important. There was no situation where there was a need for help, and parents were in the vicinity and capable of helping but did not do so. Other respondents obviously felt that, had their parents been alive, around or capable, they would have been helping out, particularly with household maintenance:

> it would be nice if they lived a bit nearer because I think my father could, perhaps, have taken a bit of the heavy work off me, you know, like gardening and decorating, anything like that. (Mrs Ord, carer)

> if my dad had still been alive I wouldn't have been doing garden now, my dad would have done all that for us . . . (Mrs Ibstock, carer)

There was a strong feeling from the interviews of both carers and spouses that their parents were, or could have been, a more acceptable source of help than were their offspring. Except when parents were frail or impoverished themselves (see below) neither carers nor spouses expressed the same degree of reluctance to accept or ask for help from their parents as they did with regard to their children. For example, Mrs Ibstock's reluctance to let her children see the level of their father's need for help has been described earlier. It was obvious from his interview that this reluctance was very strong in Mr Ibstock as well, and it was this, as much as any feelings of her own, that made her keep their children at a distance. Yet, as we have just seen, Mr Ibstock apparently had little difficulty in letting his own parents help him, even with quite intimate tasks.

Research on children caring for their elderly parents has shown how difficult it can be to reverse the 'normal' direction of care-giving between parents and offspring (e.g. Ungerson 1987). However, when disability starts in old age, there is nonetheless an expectation, not always mutual, that children will take on caring responsibilities. By contrast, when disability starts before old age carers and spouses may look more easily to their parents for help. However, this source of support is self-limiting. When parents die or become too frail to continue providing support the carer and spouse may feel that it is still too early to expect their own offspring to play a supporting role – they still 'have their own lives to lead'.

Why other relatives do or do not help

As with help from offspring, help from other relatives was influenced by distance from the respondents and other responsibilities: '. . . [wife] comes from a very big family, she has six brothers and two sisters . . . one of her sisters lives in M. so she can't come and help very much, her other sister has four children, she's running around from schools and nurseries and things like that all day . . .' (Mr Jefferson, carer). In total, two-thirds of respondents said that all or some of their other relatives were either too far away to help or had too much to do with their own families to be available to help.

Well over a half of respondents said that their other relatives, usually parents, were too elderly or frail to help. As we saw above, the frailty or ill-health of parents could represent a significant loss of potential help. Frail or ill relatives could also mean additional work for some carers and spouses:

> when my dad died my mum had to shift into a sheltered home . . . and if she's ever bad she just picks up the phone for me. She wouldn't ask anybody down there to do anything for her and that's where I find it hard if my mum takes bad because I'm running, instead of going to work, in between the two houses. (Mrs Ibstock, carer)

Some respondents clearly felt that their relatives did not understand the impact of the disability, either on spouse or carer, and therefore did not think to offer help: 'I sometimes think people don't understand what it is like unless you've lived with it. My parents have never had anything like this, so I still think today they don't really realise what it's like. I find that with a lot of people' (Mrs Ord, carer).

Another carer, whose wife was among the most disabled spouses in the study, felt not only that his relatives did not understand the implications of the disability, but also that, to some extent, they could not be expected to do so. His words are quoted at some length because they say something fundamental about the limitations of what might be expected from relatives:

> I certainly wouldn't ask a relative [to help], it's too emotional a situation to ask a relative. *I* can put up with – *do* put up with – a tremendous amount, I couldn't expect a relative on either side . . . to be able to cope with that, or to do some of the physical requirements as well because, for obvious reasons, it's OK for me to do it but not, you know, someone else . . . I mean I've got to do manual evacuations of her bowels . . .
>
> Maybe I care too much about her and about the family, I wouldn't want to give them that responsibility, I wouldn't want to put them in, I wouldn't want to see them hurt, I don't want to see them hurt, anyway, and I know that there's a strong possibility that they might be. (Mr Jefferson, carer)

The impact of disability and caring on kinship networks

The physical limitations associated with the spouse's disability and the carer's involvement in helping his or her partner meant that couples were able to give less help to others than they perhaps felt that they should. This was an additional source of stress and, sometimes, guilt:

> if [husband] had been like any other normal man and he was still working and my mum was bad I'd be down more often and I'd be able to do more for her but I can't you see, the situation that I'm in.
>
> You see if I'd been in a big family it wouldn't have been so hard because we could have sort of taken turns but with it just being me and my brother it's sort of left up to

me. But my mum's good, she doesn't bother me unless it's really necessary. (Mrs Ibstock, carer)

The issue of sharing responsibility for elderly parents and other relatives between siblings was evident in several interviews. In some it was felt to be no bad thing that siblings had had to take on more responsibility: '. . . before he was ill [husband] did everything for [his mother], he chopped sticks, he went round every day and he looked after her, but now he can't so his other brothers have had to take a turn now, which is only fair because [husband]'s always done it' (Mrs Derby, carer).

In other cases the spouse's or carer's withdrawal from responsibility for an elderly parent was a bone of contention between siblings:

> I think my sister resents it. She thinks she's been palmed off with me mother and me father, you know. There's only the two of us so she feels that I've had it good [compared] to her. She has to come home at night and cook a meal for me dad and weekends she's got him. (Mrs. Eden, spouse)

This perceived failure to help others is important because reciprocity is an important element in maintaining helping networks (Bulmer 1986). When people are unable to *give* the help that they feel they should be giving they are correspondingly uneasy about *receiving* help. This then leads, in part at least, to the determined stance of independence to which so many of the couples clung. This independence – 'we keep ourselves to ourselves' – and the whole process by which couples came to it, contributed to a weakening of kinship (and as will be shown later, neighbourhood and friendship) networks.

Furthermore, caring and disability themselves reduced the opportunities respondents had for contact with relatives: '. . . we don't go visiting much with him being like he is. . . . if you go to somebody's house you can't very well say, "Can he lay on the floor?" ' (Mrs Gifford, carer).

In summary, this group of people who might need help and support did not, on the whole, get it from relatives. In many cases there just were no relatives alive or nearby who could help; in other cases relatives had little spare time because of the demands of their own families. Furthermore, the restrictions which disability and caring responsibilities can impose weakened what might already have been quite tenuous links between relatives. Women, particularly, felt that they could not carry out their other family obligations and the opportunities for contact with relatives were reduced.

Help from neighbours

Contact with neighbours and help provided

Another possible source of informal support for carers and disabled people and, again, one emphasized in recent policy documents, is the neighbourhood. Although one or both partners in two-thirds of couples mentioned some form of help or support from neighbours, in only one case did this run to much more than doing a small amount of shopping or providing access to a telephone. No type of help was mentioned by more than three couples and there was little help to the disabled person or with domestic tasks.

In two cases only had neighbours ever helped the disabled spouse directly; in one case a neighbour had helped in an emergency, and in the other a female neighbour came in from time to time to wash and set Mrs Eden's hair.

Several couples said that they *could* call on their neighbours, if necessary, but it was clear that the circumstances would have to be exceptional for this to happen: '. . . I wouldn't like to rely on them. No. It's a bad job if you have to rely on them. You'd be in dire straits. In a very bad way . . .' (Mr Fowey, spouse).

The reasons respondents gave for their neighbours not helping them fell into patterns broadly similar to those given for children and other relatives, although their relative importance varied.

Obviously proximity is a 'given' regarding neighbours, unless people live in isolated places and, therefore, does not affect whether or not help is potentially available in the way that it does with children or other relatives. However, geographical issues did emerge for those couples who had recently moved house or whose neighbours, whom they had known well, had moved away:

> the people next door, they've just been in a twelve month. Now they came from a different environment altogether. You know, they're not country people . . . And we just haven't hit on at all. I was sorry mind because you never know when you need a neighbour . . . (Mr Hazleton, spouse)

Couples were affected by changes of this sort in two ways. On the one hand, as with the Hazletons, couples could find their new neighbours less pleasant or helpful than their previous ones had been. On the other hand, the effects of disability and caring could restrict opportunities for establishing new networks and relationships: '. . . living round here, I'm too busy really to make friends. There seem to be a lot of young couples with babies around here or elderly people so, we just keep ourselves to ourselves really' (Mrs Ord, carer).

As Mrs Ord's comment suggests, the generation to which neighbours belonged was also an important factor in determining whether or not neighbours were available to help and whether or not respondents felt that they had anything in common with them.

Half of the couples mentioned that all or some of their neighbours were elderly. Indeed, some couples found themselves *providing* support rather than receiving it:

> It was an elderly couple on the other side of us and we found out that [laughs], we was helping *them*, they were both in their eighties and he used to come round and knock on our door . . . his wife had fallen out of bed, could we go and get her back in [laughs]. We found we was helping them, but I had to put a stop to that because, I mean, sometimes [husband] wasn't fit to go round to help so I used to have to go . . . (Mrs Clifton, carer)

Others had grown old with their neighbours who were consequently no more able to provide support than the couples were to give it.

Being older constrained the formation of new relationships because, for many, it was having young children that facilitated the growth of neighbourhood networks. Once children had grown or left home the excuse for making contacts was lost:

> once the family's grown up and left home, you get into your own environment and I think it's children that makes your relationship with neighbours more or less . . .

> But once they're grown up and married and they've moved away, I don't know, you speak but you're not . . . I never *have* been a one for going in and out of people's houses. Never *have* been all the years I've lived here. Unless I was really needed. You see . . . But me children were always welcome . . . And then I'd go and look for them and things like that, you know, or they'd come in . . . me neighbours would come in here and so on, but that was when the children were little. But since then, no, I think everybody, we're just all growing old and that's it. (Mrs Baker, carer)

The importance of young children is demonstrated vividly by Mr and Mrs Eden. Although they were in their late fifties and had moved to a new house after their three sons were grown, they had been plugged-in to a helping network because their young granddaughter started to live with them. Her father had returned home when he separated from his wife, and Mr and Mrs Eden took on much of the responsibility for her care and upbringing. The Edens thus reactivated the process outlined by Mrs Baker and had established links with neighbours who, for the most part, were a generation younger than themselves. These links were based on the grandchild, but had a spin-off in relation to help for Mrs Eden from time to time.

The crucial element in all this, however, seemed to be that Mr Eden had both the time and the opportunity to reciprocate:

> It cuts both ways, you see. If the neighbour's got anything on, she might come to me one day and say, 'Can you pick my couple [of children] up from school?', which I do and fetch back home with me and I'll keep them for another ten minutes or fifteen minutes . . . 'till she's back. So, you know, so I'm repaying anything she does if she's got any problem and I can assist her I will do at the same time. So, that makes a difference, it helps her as well. (Mr Eden, carer)

Mr Eden had been away from work for some 18 months because of his own ill-health, although he was not too restricted in what he could do; consequently he had the time to reciprocate. Mrs Eden, although very limited in her daily activities, could be left for short periods during the day and, in the evenings and weekends, had her grown son at home to help out if needed; thus, Mr Eden also had the opportunity to reciprocate.

This combination of the presence of young children, and the time and opportunity to reciprocate neighbourly help is, of course, of enormous importance in regard to couples who are young at the time of onset of disability. Those whose children are grown when the disability starts have at least had the opportunity in the past to make links with their neighbours. If they remain in the same neighbourhood, even if everyone grows old and frail together, they do, at least, retain a sense of belonging. Mr and Mrs Derby, for example, although not close to their immediate neighbours did have other neighbours who, over the many years they had lived near, had become friends. By contrast, younger married couples, when the disability starts before their dependent children have grown, may have neither time nor opportunity to make these links. This leaves them reliant on help from their family which, as we have already seen, may not always be available or forthcoming, and which is, in any case, inevitably self-limiting. Only if younger married couples can replace neighbourly networks with networks which do not necessarily depend on exact reciprocity do they stand any chance of receiving informal help from outside the family. As we shall see in the section on friends, churches seem a likely source of such non-reciprocal help.

Although age and generation influenced the viability of neighbourly networks there was another set of issues, which can be broadly defined as attitudinal, which seemed to be even more influential. Most important of these was 'keeping your-self to yourself' and notions of what constituted 'good' neighbouring (Bulmer 1986). Far from a good neighbour being someone who was concerned for one's welfare and who helped out from time to time, a good neighbour for most of the respondents in this study was one who respected boundaries:

> I don't really believe in neighbouring. I like to be friendly, swap books, anything like that, but not to really get involved because I don't think it works anyway, people have got their own lives haven't they? (Mrs Derby, carer)

> I've been here 17 years and I've never asked any of the neighbours to do anything for us, definitely not. I mean I've got good neighbours, they don't come in, they don't bother you, and I don't go in there . . . (Mrs Ibstock, carer)

The price paid for this form of good neighbouring was, however, that neighbours did not understand either the spouse's disability or the effects it had on the carer. This could sometimes lead to hurtful comments and behaviour:

> it's no good relying on anybody, it's just a case of getting on wi' it yourself; make best on it, and it works out best even though we do get talked about him being a maling-erer, but . . .
> See people don't realise once door's shut, what you have to put up with, so they've just got their own problems, they think they're hard done to enough but they don't realise how other half live . . . (Mrs Gifford, carer)

Mr Jefferson had been the focus of hurtful comments from neighbours when he took responsibility for domestic tasks:

> there are certain things that . . . it's sort of OK for women to do and is a little bit frowned upon if a man does it, like hanging the washing out. *I* don't *mind* doing that at all, but there are people that think, . . . they come out with remarks like, 'You'll make somebody a good wife', which is a bit snide and a bit nasty . . .

> a neighbour, a lady near where we lived in the other house, she said 'When I see you hanging the washing out . . . I thought, well you don't hang socks that way, you don't hang dresses that way', and I said, 'So what? So I hang them out the only way that I know' and [I] says, 'If you don't mind me saying so, you didn't come across and say, "Well I'll show you how to do this", or "can I give you a hand".' [She said] 'No, I don't suppose I did.' I said, 'Well without being rude the dresses and socks [laugh] will have to stay the way they are' . . .

In some instances boundaries were kept deliberately high because of a wish to protect the spouse:

> *Interviewer: You don't get any [help] from neighbours . . . friends?*
> No, he wouldn't let them . . .
> In fact he gets so embarrassed that *I* have to do it. First thing on a morning he says, 'Put me socks on, put me slippers on, before anybody comes in'. He doesn't like to think that anybody knows what I have to do for him you see. (Mrs Baker, carer)

Mr Baker confirmed this reluctance in his own interview. He said that he would prefer to sleep in his clothes rather than have a neighbour come round to help him should it happen that his wife were ill or away.

Mrs Ibstock was also protecting her husband from the neighbours: '. . . the woman next door . . . she's a nurse, but I've never yet gone round for [her]. I've struggled myself to get him in the bath and to get him out the bath and dry him down and that because he won't have anybody else in you see'.

We see here, then, powerful attitudinal factors, centred around notions of the nature of neighbouring and the need to protect spouses, which acted as major disincentives to neighbours becoming involved with help to disabled people within marriage. Yet again, the evidence of the interviews poses a challenge to current assumptions about the nature of natural helping networks.

Help from friends

So far we have considered the help that was available to carers and spouses from what might be termed the traditional networks of family and neighbours. However, as Abrams has suggested, there is a third possible source of help and support, and one which for some groups may be more important than the neighbourhood. Beyond close kin relationships, he argued, 'our strongest bases of informal social care are those of the non-located moral communities associated with churches, races, friendship groups and certain occupational groups – *not neighbourhoods*. Neighbours and local communities come a very poor third' (Abrams 1980: 16, original emphasis).

To what extent did the carers and spouses in this study experience help from these alternative bases?

Just over a half of the carers and a half of the spouses mentioned receiving some form of practical or emotional support from friends. However, only five couples mentioned receiving anything approaching substantial or regular forms of support. Even amongst those couples who reported several sorts of help given, little of it was much beyond normal friendly helping and none was related to helping the disabled person directly. Help with transport and doing shopping or running errands were the most often mentioned types of help among the whole group. However, it seemed that knowing friends were available and would help out if necessary was as important to many people as was any help that was actually being provided:

> we have some good friends down in chapel, definitely and . . . there's two or three of them that if I wanted anything I would just need to phone them and they would come. (Mrs Hazleton, carer)

> the closest friend I've got is my daughter's godmother and she's got four children of her own so, I mean, she's tied up, if ever I did need her she would be here, lock, stock and barrel, she'd be down here like a flash, no hesitations . . . (Mrs Picton, spouse)

Similarly, and related, the experience of belonging which friendship brought with it was as important to some respondents as practical help.

In at least six cases it appeared that neither carer nor spouse had anyone whom they could really call a friend who lived within calling distance. For one couple, the multiplicity of sons and daughters, their partners and children was a clear alternative to friends. A second couple had always been fairly exclusive, relying on one another for company, and a third couple had lost friends as a result of moving house. However, the other three had all lost friends soon after the spouse became disabled:

> we used to have a lot of friends, they used never to be away, but since he came out of work four years ago most of the friends have dropped off. (Mrs Ibstock, carer).

> I found when my husband went in the wheelchair we didn't really have a lot of friends, but what friends we had disappeared quick. (Mrs Ord, carer)

> Before [accident] happened we used to have friends over, go to parties, maybe to the British Legion to a dance or . . . I'm a member of the British Legion and I've had friends there and all but, after it happened they all went their own way. I miss them. (Mr Keighley, spouse)

Some of these couples were also relatively poorly supported – either through choice or circumstance – by kinship or neighbourhood networks, leaving them particularly isolated.

Why friends do and do not help

The factors which encouraged helping relationships with friends seemed much clearer than they did with neighbours. The first of these was church membership.

For about half of those couples who had any friends at all, church or chapel membership was an important point of contact. For example, Mrs Clifton had started to attend both the local church and local chapel in the previous five or six years, since her husband had become particularly reliant on her and had made several friends at both places. Both provided her with a social life and the occasional half-day outing, and the church or chapel friends made up a helping network.

The couple who had received the most substantial help from friends, the Quincy's, had done so primarily via their church:

> We got plenty of support from friends . . . they couldn't really have given us any more really, apart from wait on us hand and foot and in our own house as servants but they practically did that too, near enough, they were very good, they couldn't have really helped any more. (Mr Quincy, carer)

Belonging to a church or a particular faith has been identified as important in maintaining the morale of carers in other settings (e.g. among the parents of children with cystic fibrosis, Burton 1975) but the argument there has tended to be that it is some aspect of having faith that contributes to this effect. More prosaically, Abrams has pointed to the preponderance of Christian helpers in 'Good Neighbour' schemes, suggesting that religion acts as an enabling factor in informal care perhaps 'as an alternative – to practical competence in providing a basis of legitimacy and confidence from which to act' (Bulmer 1986: 234).

These couple's experiences suggest two things which made religion – or rather, belonging to a church – important. First were the opportunities it provided for social contacts in the otherwise restricted social world which carers and spouses inhabited. Female carers, in particular, seemed to be freed to participate in social activities by the purposefulness or usefulness which accrued to such activities because they were associated with the church. Mrs Hazleton had been away from her home without her husband for the first time in 27 years of married life because she went as a helper on a church youth organization trip to London. She would not have done this under any other circumstances. Such social activities inevitably brought closer relationships with other people which, in time, led to the growth of friendship networks with helping potential.

Secondly, and related, it seems that church membership may allow the suspension or realignment of the expectations of reciprocity and mutual exchange on which friendship (and neighbouring) usually depend (Bulmer 1987). We have seen throughout this chapter how difficult most respondents found it to accept help offered to them or to ask for it, even from those who were very close to them. Much has been written about the influence of reciprocity and exchange on informal networks and other studies have shown that most carers find it difficult to accept help because they feel that they cannot reciprocate in similar vein (Glendining 1983; Bulmer 1986; 1987). Evidence from this study suggests that membership of a church, of itself, allows people to accept help that they perhaps would not accept in other circumstances. The Hazletons and Quincys, particularly, seemed to demonstrate that their input into the church or chapel – being members, participating in church groups and so on – made accepting practical help from other church members less problematic.

Mrs Quincy gave the clearest articulation of the belief or expectation that membership of a church gave access to help which one did not necessarily feel *had* to be reciprocated in similar kind; being a member was enough: '. . .we are Jehovah's Witnesses so they are from our religion, so they help us tremendously like that.' Of course, religion was important to these respondents in spiritual ways as well. Here, however, we have seen how important were the non-reciprocating networks which came with church membership, for those who had them.

Reciprocity was important in other circumstances as well and several respondents mentioned this when talking about help they received from their friends. Although they were no more able to reciprocate help from friends than they were that from neighbours, people clearly felt more at ease about the former source of help than about the latter. This seemed to be because a time element existed in relation to reciprocity between friends, but not between neighbours (cf. Duck 1983). Thus, some respondents felt relatively happy about accepting help from friends when they had been able to do something for those friends in the *past*: '. . . they've turned towards us in the past – not that we've been able to help financially but I've been able to help in other ways and that's made me feel better, that I'm not useless, you know. I can help somebody else out' (Mr Quincy, carer).

Others explained help from friends in terms of a return for *their* help to the community or neighbourhood more generally:

> I was the same [helpful to others] before I was bad. I'd run about after old people, deliver things to the door, off the farm. Me mate had a farm and I used to get it all for free and I used to take it to the pensioners for free – I used to be running about 20 hours a day and I enjoyed it, I enjoyed it. (Mr Baker, spouse)

> there's always somebody [friends to help]. Mind you, we've always been the same with other people you know. (Mr Derby, spouse)

Thus, people used ideas of reciprocity to 'explain' why friends helped them out but also, and perhaps more importantly, used them to justify to themselves why it was all right to accept help, such as it was, from these friends.

As with family and neighbours, friends' own family commitments and problems were seen as legitimate excuses for their not helping. Ill-health among the peers of the couples at the top end of the age range was, not surprisingly, an important constraint.

For younger respondents, their friends' child care responsibilities limited the help they could give. Responsibilities for other members of the friends' families also reduced their ability to help: '. . . [wife] has her friend, her friend lives over there, but you see *her* mother's pretty bad and she goes down a lot to her mother's which is down the bottom end and she has her hands tied three-quarters of the time' (Mr Fowey, spouse).

In all, however, these sorts of issues were cited less frequently as reasons why friends did not help out than they were when neighbours or relatives were being discussed. It is not immediately clear why this should be; perhaps respondents simply felt less need to explain or justify their friends' lack of involvement than they did their relatives. Certainly less explanation in general went on when they were talking about their friends' help.

Several people, particularly carers, felt that their circumstances since the onset of the spouse's disability had weakened friendship ties. Not being able to get out was a major consideration for both carers and spouses:

> I have no one particular friend to go about with – I mean that's pointless because she'd have to stay in like I did [laughs]. (Mrs Baker, carer)

> people'd go to town with their friends and things like that. I mean I just don't, not when he's off [work]. I mean I might do it when he's working, might just get out that bit more. And then you get . . . you see 'cos you haven't done it for so long you don't want to do it, if you know what I mean. You don't . . . it's hard just to pick up pieces where you left off so you just don't start it. So if I go to town it's usually on my own . . . (Mrs Gifford, carer)

> there isn't really *any* opportunities to make contact with any one because I'm stuck here all day and everyone else is out there all day. There's no opportunity there. (Mr Ord, spouse)

The eventual outcome of not being able to get out was that couples might 'drop out' of their previous friendship networks:

> I mean we have dropped out. We've had to drop out. What can I say? We used to do – the social groups – but at the same time, some of those friends that we had before, they're still in contact. They maybe phone us up and say, 'We'll pop over on Sunday', which is nice. (Mrs Keighley, carer)

While not being with friends as often as in the past could be painful for couples, being in contact could also sometimes cause sorrow as the past was compared with the present:

> You adjust yourself. You find you are adjusting whether you like it or whether you don't. It's only when you're in contact with friends the same age as yourself, and, er . . .
>
>   They're out and about in the car and away and all the rest of it and we're . . . these things don't happen. (Mrs Keighley, carer)

Finally, as we have already seen, friendships were sometimes put under strain by friends not fully understanding the spouse's disability or being afraid of it in some way.

Again, then, we find that a possible source of informal help and support to carers and spouses was not, except in a few cases, functioning as such. More than half of the couples had experienced a weakening of friendships after the spouse had become disabled either because they could no longer participate in activities with their friends or because their friends had withdrawn. Thus, the opportunities for friendship networks to provide practical help and emotional support were reduced.

Conclusions

Other studies of disability and of informal care have shown how little relatives outside the nuclear family unit, neighbours or friends become involved in helping disabled people when they already have a carer. This chapter has examined the actual provision of help and support from these sources, and has explored the factors which can facilitate or militate against informal help giving. As in other studies we have seen that informal help to households where a carer is already present is limited.

A set of conditions has to be met before members of any informal network *can* help. They must live relatively near, they must have adequate financial or quasi-financial resources to enable them to carry out their wish to help, and they must be sufficiently healthy to be able to help. The interviews showed clearly that most of these younger couples had few network members who met all these conditions. Beyond this, however, there was a complex set of structural and attitudinal factors which constrained both the provision and acceptability of informal support.

Parents believed, and with some justification, that their offspring had enough to do bringing up their own children, holding down paid work, and dealing with their own problems. Carers and their spouses actively chose not to rely on their children for help, either because they felt that it would be unfair to do so or because, in a few cases, they would be unhappy if their children were ever to discover what was needed in the way of help to the spouse.

Similarly, respondents wanted to keep their problems and needs from their neighbours. This was because, first, they did not feel it appropriate that their neighbours *should* know and, secondly, because they felt it even less appropriate that neighbours should help beyond providing normal neighbourly services.

Furthermore, some spouses and carers had little opportunity, time or energy to build up and maintain neighbourly and friendship networks. Even family networks and previously strong friendships could atrophy. By definition, then, many of these couples had weak, or weakening, informal networks. The issue of reciprocity was vitally important here and the analysis shows how couples got (and received) help most readily when they had the opportunity to reciprocate, or when they belonged to networks where some suspension of the normal expectations of reciprocity and mutual exchange was possible, or when help given to them now could be interpreted as a return for help they gave to others in the past.

In sum, many of this group of carers and disabled people had only residual or in some cases no networks of family, friends and neighbours which did or could help them. Even where networks existed respondents were not at all keen that these *should* be used to help. Policies based on assumptions that informal networks can or should be depended upon for help and support to disabled people and their carers are likely to leave the needs of married couples – and other groups – largely unmet.

C H A P T E R

Help from forma[...] services

Introduction

A series of reports in the recent past has criticized the availability of services for younger physically disabled people, and those who help and support them on an unpaid basis (Beardshaw 1988; Fiedler 1988; Edwards and Warren 1990). Beardshaw calls these services the 'cinderella of cinderella services' (p. 7) and points to substantial inadequacies

> both of quantity and quality: not only are levels of provision inadequate, but the right *kind* of services – ones which would enable disabled people to be autonomous and which minimise the burden on carers – often do not exist. (Beardshaw 1988: 45, original emphasis)

These criticisms are not new ones, however. Since the mid-1960s researchers have repeatedly catalogued the lack of adequate housing, aids, adaptations, domestic, nursing and personal care services for younger physically disabled people (for example, Sainsbury 1970; Harris 1971; Blaxter 1976; Knight and Warren 1978; Locker 1983; Morris 1989; Creek *et al*. not dated).

Appropriate accommodation is one of the most important pieces in the jigsaw of provision which enables disabled people to live good quality lives in the community (Morris 1989; Dunn 1990). Despite this, housing is a topic that is all but ignored in community care policy and practice (Oldman 1991). Evidence suggests that as recently as 1987 there were more than three-quarters of a million physically disabled people in Britain who were inadequately housed, with a shortage of around 150,000 purpose-built or adapted rented public sector dwellings (cited in Fiedler 1988).

The OPCS surveys of disability showed that around 15 per cent of younger disabled people had had to move from previous accommodation 'because of their disability' (Martin *et al*. 1989: table 8.3). In fact, as subsequent questions in the survey revealed, disabled people had to move not so much because of their disability as because their existing housing was inadequate for their needs. Steps and stairs were major problems. Overall, 31 per cent of all disabled people (including older ones) felt that their present housing was inadequate. Again steps and stairs were major problems.

ch also reveals substantial problems with the supply of aids and adap-
s which could make otherwise inadequate housing more suitable. Long
ys in the supply of aids or carrying out of adaptations, restricted local auth-
rity budgets, people being asked to contribute more than they feel that they can
afford, and the provision of aids and adaptations which do not suit the individual
are all described in the literature. An issue which is of particular relevance for the
research on which this book is based is the tendency of standard adapted or
specially built housing to be designed with disabled *men* who have non-disabled
wives in mind (Locker 1983).

Services such as domiciliary care (home help) and community nursing services
also create difficulties for younger disabled people. Generally speaking, service
provision in the community serves predominantly to support disabled or older
people who do not have resident carers (Arber *et al.* 1988; Green 1988; Parker
1990; Parker and Lawton 1992). This is particularly the case with services which
are domestic in nature, for example, home helps and meals-on-wheels.

Younger physically disabled adults are far less likely to receive community
services than other groups (Beardshaw 1988), again particularly when they live
with other adults, especially spouses (Fiedler 1988). Professionals tend to assume
that the provision of domestic or personal help will present no problems to those
who have partners. Despite the fact that it is women who generally provide
domestic and personal care services to others, professionals seem particularly
blind to the needs of younger disabled women for assistance (Blaxter 1976). As a
consequence, spouses may have to give up paid work and families become doubly
disabled as both home-making and breadwinning capacities are reduced (Blaxter
1976; Morris 1989).

Even when younger physically disabled people do receive services, there are
questions about the quality and, increasingly, the appropriateness of these. Particular difficulties arise over frequency and timing. Community nursing services,
for example, which disabled people may need to get them up and dressed in the
morning, are often unable to guarantee nurses arriving at a given time and,
moreover, at a time which meets the disabled person's needs. As a result, relatives
or friends may take over personal care that would otherwise be provided by a
nurse (Morris 1989). Domestic help, too, may not be as younger disabled people
want it. Younger women who consider themselves responsible for the domestic
arrangements of their household want help to be provided in the form *they* want
it, not as local authority guidelines, trade union guidance or the idiosyncrasies of
the particular home help determine (Blaxter 1976; Locker 1983; Morris 1989).
Taking away a home-maker's right to decide how her household is run can be just
as destructive of self-esteem as taking away a main earner's right to earn.

Inadequate and inappropriate support services are not just an issue for disabled
people. As the above suggests, they can mean that relatives, friends and neighbours of disabled people may be drawn into providing unpaid help. In the total
absence of services, the help of informal services may be all that stands between a
disabled person and residential care. When available services are of a poor quality
or inappropriate to the disabled person's desired lifestyle, informal carers may be
the only way in which the disabled person can lead the sort of life that he or she
wishes. However, as Morris (1989) points out, this interdependence can bring
mixed feelings with it: 'We have complicated feelings about receiving help; on

the one hand helpers can bring about independence, on the other hand their very necessity can make us feel helpless and dependent' (Morris 1989: 42).

Furthermore, as Brisenden (cited by Morris 1991: 164) has suggested, dependence on a relative or partner can be 'the most exploitative of all forms of so-called care delivered in our society for it exploits both the carer and the person receiving care. It ruins relationships between people and results in thwarted life opportunities on both sides of the caring equation.'

As we saw in Chapter 2, disabled people have argued increasingly for adequately financed and self-directed care arrangements to be available for all with care needs. However, as was discussed in that chapter, this model is not without its problems for married couples, where the ability to exercise choice and self-direction may be influenced by factors other than disability.

In the remainder of this chapter we will be looking at the services which couples in the study did or did not receive. Local authority services, community-based health services, hospital discharge and continuing care, and voluntary organizations are all included. We will also look at why people received so little help and at what else they would have liked to receive. We start by looking at help provided by the local authority.

Local authority services

Aids, adaptations and housing

Just over half of the couples had received some form of practical help from their local authority, usually the social services department, ranging from a car badge only to extensive help with adaptations and alterations to the home. Six couples had been provided with aids to daily living free of charge, the majority of which were used for bathing or toileting, while eight had had some adaptation or alteration to their homes which had been carried out or funded, either wholly or in part, by the local authority. These were more diverse in their nature and objectives than were the aids, ranging from ramps and stair rails, through major adaptations to kitchens and bathrooms, to the installation of lifts. However, no disabled spouse was wholly independent of his or her partner's help as a result of aids or adaptations.

The couple with the highest level of provision were the Ibstocks. They had a platform lift from their living room to the bedroom, stair rails, a raised toilet seat, a bath stool and rail, and external rails by the front door. Their house was a council property and they had not had to make any financial contribution.

By contrast, at the lowest level of provision, the Keighley's had no provided aids at the time of the interview. They had been given a commode after Mr Keighley had the accident which damaged his back and he had been unable to manage the stairs, and a bath seat later. The couple had then been transferred to a local authority flat which was adapted for a disabled person. Some years later, after Mr Keighley's compensation claim had finally been settled (12 years after his accident), they bought a bungalow which had been built to wheelchair access standard. Bath and toilet rails were fitted as standard.

The provision of adaptations and aids, and removal to housing more suitable for the disabled spouse had been alternative options for some couples. For example, Mr and Mrs Ibstock had contacted the social services department about a year after Mr Ibstock had left work when his multiple sclerosis was having a substantial affect on his physical abilities. Their social worker had discussed the possibility of moving from their local authority, semi-detached house to a ground floor flat. The Ibstocks were not keen to do this; they had lived in the house for 17 years and had done a lot of work to it over the years, they did not want to move to an area they did not know and which might not be as pleasant as the one they currently lived in, and they did not want to lose any bedrooms as that would mean that their grandchildren could not stay with them. The social worker consequently arranged for a fairly substantial programme of alterations and adaptations, and the provision of various aids which enabled Mr Ibstock to get about the house and upstairs. Mrs Ibstock felt that they had been very fortunate: 'Well I think we are fortunate because he's got his lift and that in, if he didn't have that in I don't think we could stay here and he likes it here . . .'.

Some couples had been offered little option but to move into already adapted or purpose-designed accommodation, but this had quite striking effects on their neighbourhood networks. The Keighleys had been moved into what Mr Keighley considered a rough area and one which contained many pensioners. The Jeffersons had been similarly catapulted into an older and labelled generation, when they sold their terraced house and moved into a local authority bungalow:

> if we had a more mixed community where there were able bodied and disabled
> people together . . . I don't think that it is a good idea to separate particular areas as if
> to say that's where the disabled people live. (Mr Jefferson, carer)

Removal had not always meant that the disabled spouse's needs were met. The Verwoods had been moved to a house with a larger living room so that Mrs Verwood could sleep downstairs! Nine years later a stair lift was fitted, rather to the Verwoods' surprise, and Mrs Verwood was able to see the upper storey of her home for the first time and start to sleep in the same room as her husband again. Similarly, the Jeffersons had moved into more suitable housing, but the local authority still had to adapt the kitchen and bathroom, fit a shower and sliding doors, and install hoists in the bathroom and bedroom after they moved in. The only ways in which the accommodation had been suitable at the outset was that it had a ramp to the front door, was all on one level, and had sufficient bedrooms for the couple and their sons.

The issue of money and access to appropriate housing was crucially important to several of the couples, not just those who had had adaptations or who had moved. The ability or inability of those who were not local authority tenants to purchase appropriate accommodation or adapt their existing home substantially affected the quality of life of both carers and spouses.

Home help, day care and other services

Only two couples, the Jeffersons and the Verwoods, received home help services; in both cases the disabled spouse was a woman. In the same two couples the spouses also attended a local authority day centre. One other couple had an orange sticker car badge although this was, in fact, for the carer rather than the spouse. This was the only help they had had from their social services department and they appeared to have little need for other help at that time. Finally, one spouse mentioned the welfare rights advice and help that he had received via a social worker who, among other things, had actively helped him with a claim for mobility allowance.

Access to help from the local authority

Only two couples had any current, regular contact with a key-worker who could help the carer or spouse negotiate for services; in both cases this was a community nurse (see later). Other couples had, in the past, had times when they had been in regular contact with a social worker, but this contact had often ceased when aids and alterations had been organized or a crisis had passed. In some cases social workers who had left were not replaced.

This lack of regular contact with a social worker or other key-worker often left the onus with the carer or spouse to identify needs and make an approach:

> it's like I said to me friends, we don't want people on our doorstep all the time, but it would be nice to feel now and again that someone is interested. Well, you'd think now and again, with him being on disabled all these years someone would, you know, just come and see if he was all right. (Mrs Clifton, carer)

When disabled people and carers do not have regular contact with a key worker, access to services depends crucially on their knowledge that such services exist and, beyond that, on perceived eligibility (Kerr 1983). Even when eligibility is recognized, services may not be taken up because the individual, for various reasons, prefers to 'manage' or because the services on offer are seen as inappropriate. All these factors were evident here, leading to situations where couples had paid for aids or adaptations themselves when they might have received help, where they had waited for longer than was necessary to receive help, and where, at the time of the interview, they had long standing needs for help which were unlikely to be met without substantial intervention from an outsider (see below).

Community health services

Community nursing

Seven couples in the study had received help via the community nursing services at some stage, but at the time of the interviews only three were in regular contact. One couple was receiving daily visits from a district nurse to dress the spouse's wound; another couple received a weekly visit during which the district nurse gave the spouse a bedbath and checked (and if necessary changed) her bladder catheter; and another couple received weekly check-up visits. This last couple had also been supplied with a portable hoist and a hospital bed through the community health services. Two others were in contact for incontinence supplies only.

Of the four spouses with the most serious impairments (and most heavily involved carers) only one received help from the community nursing services with personal care – and that only once a week. Although grateful for the general surveillance which the district nurse also provided, Mr Jefferson clearly did not feel that her weekly visits made any significant difference to him:

> She'll come and . . . she'll dress her, just similar things to what I do . . . she'll check
> her catheter and things like that . . . and then she gives her a bed bath on the bed,
> but I've got to be there with [wife] not being able to stand at all, I've got to lift her,
> the nurse won't lift her, so I've got to be there anyway.

It seemed highly likely that had Mrs Jefferson not had a catheter fitted then there would not have been even this weekly visit.

Mr Selsdon also had weekly visits from a nurse, again to check on his general condition and on his catheter. After Mr Selsdon had had his second leg amputated and before Mrs Selsdon had been supplied with a portable hoist, district nurses had been visiting three times a day. Since the arrival of the hoist, however, Mrs Selsdon had received no help with caring tasks. Moreover, the equipment Mrs Selsdon had been given was both old and badly designed for her situation. The hospital bed she had been provided with created particular difficulties:

> you can see the height of that when I'm washing him, I'm on tip-toe reaching over
> the back . . . As far as I can see, what happens is when you need equipment like that
> in the house, they give you what they won't use in the hospital. And yet, if you look
> at it another way, if you're willing to look after people at home, you're saving them
> hundreds of pounds a week if you can believe what they say what it costs to keep
> people in hospitals and things. So why can't we have decent equipment? I mean
> that's what you get, you know, what's obsolete as far as the hospitals are concerned.
> (Mrs Selsdon, carer)

Mr Derby also had regular visits from a district nurse for attention to a large wound. This had been going on for over three years at the time of the interview. Mrs Derby played a large part in this process; she acted as 'dirty' nurse when the district nurse irrigated and dressed the wound in the morning, and was solely responsible for the dry dressing applied in the evening. Mrs Derby had always assumed that her role in this was important to Mr Derby's recovery and was surprised that, when she entered hospital herself, the district nurse did not visit again in the evening:

> I thought if it's important that I do it in the evening then surely when I'm not there
> they will do it, but they didn't. And . . . well, they must know what they're doing,
> they must have thought it was going to be all right.

It is not surprising that this incident led Mrs Derby to wonder, if the evening dressing was not that necessary, why she did it anyway, but she had never questioned the district nurse or anyone else about this.

The general practitioner

Given the high proportion of spouses in the study whose impairments were caused by or associated with chronic ill health (see appendix) one might have expected that the general practitioner would have played an important role in couples' lives, at the very least as a gatekeeper to other services. However, while some couples saw their GP regularly and relied on him or her for help and advice, there were as many who rarely saw their GP or, if they did, felt that they received little help or advice.

One of the most important elements of a good relationship with a GP was his or her responsiveness and availability: 'When I was very depressed . . . she was available for me twenty-four hours a day. She made herself available. She told me that and she wanted to see me . . .' (Mrs Quincy, spouse).

By contrast, a poor relationship with a GP was often characterized as one in which the GP had no time for the individual, did not know or understand the situation, or merely wrote prescriptions. This was particularly the case for carers:

sometimes I have trouble with my back and the only comment if I go to the doctor's about it, he says, 'Well, that's a nurse's occupational hazard' and he'd give us some tablets and, you know, 'See what they do' . . . (Mr Jefferson, carer)

Several of the spouses, although they felt that they had a reasonable relationship with the doctor, were reluctant to contact him or her regularly, often because they felt there was little the doctor could do for them or because their condition was outside the general practitioner's expertise.

While it was true that GPs could do little for most of the spouses in terms of curing or ameliorating their condition, a few clearly took a lot of interest and cared deeply about their patients' and, sometimes, the carers' situation.

[He is] the most kindest man – he's only a young man. He's young, very, very, young and even through the court case [compensation claim] he was very helpful, very helpful. All the time I've been ill he attends me. (Mr Keighley, spouse)

Mr Keighley was clearly overwhelmed by the quality and extent of attention he received from his GP. During a particularly critical time the GP had visited every day, including the weekends, for three weeks. He counselled Mr Keighley about the couple's sexual difficulties and he allowed Mr Keighley to ventilate his anger:

I've just got to get it out and I pick on her and the doctor said, 'She's your ally, the one you can depend on, and you take it out on her and you shouldn't, 'cos she's your main ally and she'll stand by you, whether it's good or bad, up or down, she's always there beside you', he said, 'and think yourself lucky' . . . 'Don't take it out on her, take it out on me . . . . it won't hurt me what you call me but it will hurt [wife], hurt her deeply, but it won't hurt me, I couldn't care a jigger what you say to me . . .' And this made me calm down a lot, it made me ashamed of myself, you know. But he did get the message home to me, in a nice [way]. He's only young. (Mr Keighley, spouse)

Younger and/or women doctors seemed particularly likely to have been supportive for spouses. Mr Ord, who had become disabled because of post-operative complications (see below), had found his young GP's honesty and openness with him refreshing:

They [hospital] offered me anti-depressants because sometimes I get a bit gloomy . . . but I asked my own GP his opinion, and I quite like my own GP, in fact, as the medical profession goes, he's not bad – and he said – in his opinion I didn't want anti-depressants because, to put it bluntly, he said, 'Well, in your position you're entitled to get pissed off' . . . (Mr Ord, spouse)

These GPs had encouraged their patients to apply for various disablement benefits, had referred them on to social services departments and other service providers, and kept a watching brief when there was nothing else they could do.

Obviously, this handful of doctors worked to a model of general practice that was near to ideal for their disabled patients. However, they were a minority.

Moreover, although their practice with the spouses was so good, there was a suspicion that this could occasionally blind them to the carers' needs. Mrs Ord, for example, had once fallen off her moped and cracked some ribs. She could hardly move herself and certainly could not move Mr Ord up and down stairs, and in and out of the bath. The GP had visited and offered to get a district nurse in. However, *Mr* Ord refused the suggestion and the GP did not challenge him. This was a situation in which the disabled spouse's views should have been challenged and the GP was the only one with the power to do so.

Hospital discharge and the continuity of professional care

All the couples in the study, both carers and spouses, had some experience of hospital in-patient and out-patient services. While many respondents had much to say about their experiences of hospital care, what follows is about those aspects of these experiences which impinged directly on their home lives. The issue of discharge from hospital was the most important of these.

The time of discharge from a hospital can be one of great stress for both the ex-patient and his or her family. Even if the patient has been looking forward to returning home there can still be great anxiety about the sudden loss of 24-hour professional care; this is particularly the case when the patient is still rather ill when sent home. On the carer's side there may be anxieties about how she or he will cope and, again, these anxieties are more acute when the patient is still quite ill or needing a lot of help. There were several examples in the study where couples felt that the spouse had been discharged from hospital too early or that adequate support had not been available in the community at the time of discharge. In addition, one carer felt that her husband should have been admitted to hospital when his drug treatment was altered.

Mr Ord had been sent home from hospital in the middle of winter, unable to stand, and with no apparent provision for surveillance from the community medical or nursing services:

> after about a week [after husband's discharge from hospital] I was just in tears at our
> GP's then . . . I just said, I just can't do it, I can't get him out of the bed. And he got
> me a nurse round and she showed me how to get him out of bed and that was it,
> nobody else ever came after that.

In fact, because Mrs Ord was unable to leave her husband after he returned home they had improvised for some days using milk bottles and kitchen bowls in place of a urine bottle and a bed-pan. The swelling of Mr Ord's leg and the deep vein thrombosis which caused it went undetected for at least two weeks.

Other cases were less dramatic but created no less cause for concern. Mr Keighley, for example, had been able to do so little for himself when he left hospital that Mrs Keighley had given up her job, 'on doctor's orders'.

However, it was not only the discharge of spouses from hospital that caused problems. *Carers* had also been in hospital and sent home with little or nothing in the way of support. Mrs Derby, for example, had undergone major abdominal surgery:

Interviewer: Were you offered any extra help at home [when discharged]?

No . . . you see they couldn't throw me out quick enough . . . the day before they came round and said, 'You can go home now', but I said, 'It isn't as easy as that. In my case I can't just ring my husband and say fetch me. For one thing we've got no transport, for another thing my husband can't anyway, so I just can't arrange anything until I can get my son and daughter to arrange something'. So reluctantly he said, 'Well, do this as quickly as possible because we need the bed', which makes you feel awful really doesn't it? (Mrs Derby, carer)

Mrs Derby was sent home with instructions not to do the vacuum cleaning or any lifting, but with no domestic help she had no option but to do some. Possibly as a result of this, she started bleeding internally and had to be re-admitted to hospital: 'Obviously when I came out, under the circumstances, I couldn't have the convalescence that you really need, when you've got somebody to look after, can you?'

Similarly, Mrs Ibstock had been told not to lift anything when she left hospital, also after major abdominal surgery. In this case the hospital was aware of Mrs Ibstock's responsibilities for her husband and she had been asked if she needed help. The combination of her pride and the knowledge that Mr Ibstock would not like to be cared for by outsiders made her say no. As with the Ords' GP when Mrs Ord cracked her ribs, this seemed to be an occasion when professional advice should possibly have over-ruled the spouse's reluctance to accept help.

The third carer who had this sort of experience was Mr Quincy. He had contracted meningitis and had almost died. Not only was he unable to care for his wife when he was sent home, he was himself still in the throes of the illness:

The hospital discharged me very early actually and [the GP] was very annoyed about that. I should have been in hospital for at least three weeks to a month – I was so bad, but they discharged me after a week and the day they discharged me I was vomiting violently and I couldn't walk properly, just couldn't keep myself steady, I just had no balance, no control and that was what I was like when they discharged me, so as regards professional help you can forget it. (Mr Quincy, carer)

Mrs Quincy, who had osteo-arthritis of the spine, hip and shoulder, had two young children to look after at the same time as Mr Quincy. A short while later their son was admitted to hospital with pneumonia. It is not surprising, perhaps, that soon after Mr Quincy recovered Mrs Quincy had a nervous breakdown.

All of a sudden, you know, I mean I'd coped with [the disability and illnesses] all the years and accepted . . . well, I'd say accepted, I've accepted some of them. And when more and more come – I just didn't want to – it was as if I'd had enough, you know. I didn't want any more. (Mrs Quincy, spouse)

In total there had been serious lapses in the continuity of care, or of communication between the hospital and community-based health services, in over half of the couples where the spouse and/or carer had ever been an in-patient. The incidence of such difficulties is worryingly high.

Voluntary organizations

There was little evidence in the study of substantial involvement in or help from voluntary organizations. Only two couples were active members of any voluntary organization (the Multiple Sclerosis Society); one other carer was a member of the Parkinson's Disease Society, but this had no local branch. Two couples had received help from Community Programme (CP) schemes, in both cases with gardening although both were anticipating future help with decorating. One couple, who also belonged to the MS Society, had received information and advice from a local independent advice agency, and another mentioned receiving a bath seat and walking-stick from a local organization 'that our doctors and volunteers run'. In total, then, fewer than a third of couples had had any contact with a voluntary organization.

Carers seemed to get more out of involvement with the voluntary societies than did the spouses. In all these cases spouses had been resistant to involvement, at least initially:

> We went along [to the local MS Society] and that takes a little bit of doing because not everybody can – [wife] was still walking at that time, not everybody can go into a room where there's a lot of people in wheelchairs, depending on how badly affected they are. 'Cos they're going to say, 'I'm going to end up like that'. On the other hand you could say, 'Well thank God I'm not as bad as that'. But it took [wife] quite a while · to get used to [it] . . . (Mr Jefferson carer)

Mr Ibstock had also been reluctant to become involved in the local MS society, but had eventually come round to the idea by the 'thank God I'm not as bad as that' route and had subsequently found it useful to be able to talk to others with the same condition. However, it was still clear that the carers gained most. From society booklets, talks and contacts with other members they had discovered much about the nature and likely prognosis of their spouses' condition, about sources of help, and about local services. This knowledge had obviously made these carers more confident about making contact with service providers and asking for help.

That such a relatively small input of information had made such a difference is an obvious vindication of the importance of making information easily available. It is not so clear that the best way to make information available is through voluntary organizations. Only three couples had any contact with a society and few of the other spouses had conditions or impairments with clearly identifiable labels that would lead them to similar societies. Moreover, it is obvious that not every one is keen on joining organizations and that spouses have to cross difficult psychological barriers before joining becomes acceptable to them. For some it may never become acceptable.

Accounting for unmet need for services

One of the major causes of unmet need among these couples appeared to be the failure of professionals, particularly when hospital-based, to recognize that the spouses might encounter problems at home. Consequently, respondents were not referred on to appropriate sources of help either within the hospital service itself (e.g. the hospital social worker) or outside (e.g. the local social services team or community nursing service). As we have seen, the time of discharge from hospital to the community, and lack of support at that time, was a major problem for many couples.

Some couples just did not know that they might be eligible for practical help via their local authority. This sometimes seemed to be tied up with confusion about the relative responsibilities of the DHSS (as it then was) in regard to social security and the local authority social services department. However, even among those couples who had received practical help, confusion could exist between who was responsible for aids and adaptations, and who was responsible for benefits.

Other couples did not see available help as appropriate or adequate. This was especially the case with domestic and nursing services for female carers, and with day care and respite care for spouses.

Mrs Hazleton, for example, had been offended when the only help that had been suggested for her and her husband was meals-on-wheels:

> I says, 'I don't want meals-on-wheels'. I says, 'I can cook what he wants – we don't want them'. I says, 'I can do what I want and – if that's all they can offer, they can keep it'. (Mrs Hazleton, carer)

For women carers, however, the issue of appropriateness also seemed to be related to ideas of deservingness and managing:

> things would really have to be on top of me before I would ask for home help because there's an awful lot of people can't get it at the present moment . . . So I wouldn't be very happy about a home help having to come here rather than they go to somebody in dire straits, if you like, you know, I can manage. (Mrs Keighley, carer)

> I prefer, if I can manage, I'd rather do it. I think it's wrong to tie nurses up if you can manage without. I mean, they're far better spending their time with people that can't manage. (Mrs Selsdon, carer)

By contrast, the two male carers whose wives received home help services did not see this input as inappropriate, presumably because it replaced services that their wives were no longer providing. Female carers, even when heavily involved, felt that as long as they could manage their domestic work they had no right to expect home help:

> *Interviewer: Would you have had a home help if one had been offered to you?*
> Well it has been suggested but I prefer to manage as long as I can. If I found I couldn't it would be a different matter. (Mrs Selsdon, carer)

Given that Mrs Selsdon was the most heavily involved carer, managing here seems to be quite clearly related to her assessment of her own physical condition, rather than to any assessment of the overall responsibility she was carrying.

Similar considerations seemed to be at work among service providers. Mrs Ord was another heavily involved carer, but received no help with the tasks she carried out. Yet:

> This year my wife has not been very well, she's developed colitis. And I've never seen the man who is our social worker. I spoke to him over the phone. There was a possibility my wife was going to have to go into hospital and he would have offered a home help then and my GP would have arranged for a nurse to get me up in the morning, and they would probably have arranged meals-on-wheels for about three days a week. But I don't actually get any sort of assistance from anyone [at the moment]. (Mr Ord, spouse)

There could hardly be a clearer articulation of service providers' views of the role of domestic services *vis-à-vis* female carers, or of the way in which services are provided only when the carer is unavailable, rather than to enable the disabled person to be independent of family help.

Another contributory factor to unmet need (for carers) was the negotiation that went on between the carer and the spouse about the acceptability of help from outside. We have already seen that Mr Ord refused the services of a district nurse, without consulting his wife, when she cracked her ribs. He was not the only male spouse to be reluctant or to have refused to accept help with personal care from others. Mrs Ibstock refused help when *she* returned from hospital because she felt that her husband would be uncomfortable with it. He confirmed this reluctance in his own interview:

> you're so dependent, like a little baby, dependent on someone else . . .
> Help us to the toilet, help us back from the toilet, and do things like that for you. I don't know, I felt like that with my own wife, I don't know how those people feel that haven't got a wife and have to let strangers do it. It must be terrible for them kind of people. (Mr Ibstock, spouse)

This issue came up again in relation to services which the spouse had used, but found inappropriate. Mr Ord, for example, needed stimulating and rewarding day-time occupation, although he was in too much pain to sustain full-time, paid work. Local day facilities, however, were orientated towards a much older, and perhaps more intellectually impaired, population:

> there is a day centre not so far from here, we pass it sometimes, if we're out walking. I don't know, maybe it's the wrong impression you get about it but I don't think it's a place I would like to see my husband. I feel he's a very intelligent person and I think he could do with company where he could have a good conversation with people, not put somewhere, you know, to play cards or play ping-pong or whatever, because he's not that type of person. (Mrs Ord, carer)

Mr Ord's experience of entering the local Younger Disabled Person's Unit (YDU) confirmed Mrs Ord's feelings about the inappropriateness of such provision. Mr Ord had been to the YDU twice and refused to return. He described being 'treated like a half-wit' and had attempted to buck the system:

> I know one of the things that they did in the YDU, it upset the system, I got a bollocking for it. They organised a day trip – and I refused to go, because they had a bus with . . . Spastics Society written on the side of it. And there was no way that I was going in that bus. No, there wasn't. I just wasn't going in it. [The ward sister] went bloody mad . . . (Mr Ord, spouse)

Mr Ord identified part of the problem with the unit as being that the sister in charge had previously worked in a large psychiatric hospital. He clearly felt that the values and attitudes that she brought from that experience were inappropriate to his situation and that of those like him:

> When I was last in that YDU she, the sister I'm referring to, had this idea that if you weren't playing cards you had to – I think at the time it was in August or September – had to be making bloody Christmas cards for her . . . stamp a cut-out potato on a piece of old card and say that's a Christmas card, hand-made by the YDU written on by the staff nurse, in copper plate at the back. (Mr Ord, spouse)

Mr Ord was not prepared to put up with an unsatisfactory form of help in order to give his wife a break. Mrs Ord clearly regretted this, but supported her husband's decision:

> We thought the idea was good, it gave me a break, but he wouldn't go back again because he was treated as a half-wit. You know, the body mightn't be much good, but he's quite mentally alert. So I can't really blame him for not wanting to go back. (Mrs Ord, carer)

The inappropriateness of the culture of YDUs caused problems even when spouses were prepared to use them. Mrs Jefferson had been offered respite care at a local YDU at a time when Mr Jefferson was particularly stressed. Although Mr Jefferson appreciated the break that the respite care gave him he was not entirely happy with it. Mrs Jefferson did not enjoy the experience and appeared to do little more than watch television while she was away. She was not able to lie on her bed in the afternoon, as she did at home, and found sitting in a chair all day extremely tiring. Mr Jefferson felt that his wife deteriorated physically, even in the short period she was away, and articulated the need for a much better quality of care. Mrs Jefferson, in contrast to Mr Ord, bore the experience because she felt that the break was important for her husband:

> I didn't think there's a lot of things [caring tasks] right for a man, but when they're chucked in this position, I mean there's millions like me in this country, and it's just seeing how they cope, that's why I go into hospital for two days, to give him a break.

Felt need for formal services

As well as talking about their experiences of services they had received, respondents were also asked about the help, advice or support which *they* felt they needed, both at the time the spouse became disabled or ill and at the present. They were also asked what they saw as the most difficult aspect of their current situation.

Bradshaw (1972) has argued that the difficulties of accounts of 'felt' need are that, on the one hand, perceptions of need are 'limited by the perceptions of the individual – whether they know there is a service available, as well as a reluctance in many situations to confess a loss of independence' and, on the other hand, can be 'inflated by those who ask for help without really needing it'. The reactions of the couples in this study tended much more to the former than to the latter. Indeed, around a third of carers and a quarter of spouses expressed either fatalistic views about the hope of any service ever being able to help them or a reluctance to make demands for a service. Such views seemed closely related to the length of time for which the spouse had been disabled or to the nature of his or her condition:

> Well I don't really know what help I could have had really, there's nothing anybody could have done really, is there? (Mrs Derby, carer)

> we're at such a point where we've done it that long for ourself, I just don't know what I'd want, I just don't . . . I mean I'm reluctant, if anybody came to help him because they just might not do the right thing, you see. We've just learnt ourself over years

and, like I say, I'm a bit reluctant now. You do get to a point and you get told 'no' that many times, you think it's not worth bothering with. (Mrs Gifford, carer)

This depression of the ability to acknowledge or express need – to do something about it – has also been identified by Thompson (1987), whose sample included a high proportion of spouse carers, and in studies of other types of carers (Glendinning 1985). Perhaps because of this reluctance, the needs that couples were able to identify tended to be rather modest.

Over a third of carers said that at the time when their spouses had first become disabled or ill they would have liked to have had some form of emotional support. Only one spouse talked of a similar need. This was not exclusively a gender-related issue because one of the male carers (and a male spouse) were able to say that they, too, had needed emotional support. It seemed, rather, to be closely related to the fact of being a carer and, perhaps, to the fact that the help and support available at that time tended to be directed at the spouse :

I know [the occupational nurse] comes from [husband's] work but she more or less talks to [husband], she's ever so nice but I don't actually have anybody who'll come and talk to me, hear my side on it . . . (Mrs Gifford, carer)

Emotional support at a time of crisis was associated with the need to know more about what was happening and what was likely to happen. This was a theme that ran through both carers' and spouses' accounts of their past and present needs. As well as the carers' needs for information about their spouses' prognoses, both partners mentioned the need to learn about their entitlement to benefits and for general financial advice. As Mr Mead pointed out, the period after discharge from hospital is not an ideal one for negotiating the benefits system, particularly when one has had little experience of it previously:

I think they should have somebody come round to talk to you about what's going to happen to you when you come home [from hospital] and what your finances [are] going to be . . . get it all into motion. It would save a lot of time when you come out of hospital because if you're on crutches and your leg is bandaged and your back or whatever's injured you can't get out and you can't ask your wife to do it because she's got to keep an eye on you, so it's six months to get yourself going again . . .

The need for this sort of help and advice could extend well beyond the initial period after injury or diagnosis:

I think it would be helpful if people in my situation were told what was there for them, instead of being left to plod on and find out. I mean, money isn't everything but it certainly makes life comfortable.
Interviewer: And you've missed out on a lot?
And we've missed out on it [pause] and I think, you know, my husband has enough problems without having to worry about money. (Mrs Ord, carer)

Financial issues and benefit entitlements were a considerable worry for couples; over a half mentioned money (or the lack of it) as a major problem. This issue will be dealt with in more detail in the following chapter.

The other need for information articulated by couples was for help and advice with obtaining or buying suitable equipment and on the availability of services, a finding which ties in with the lack of contact with social workers or occupational therapists:

I'd try and get some gadgets I think, but I haven't a clue where to go for them . . . I think you've got to be chronic before they'll do anything like that. (Mrs Newham, spouse)

It is not surprising that spouses were more likely than carers to articulate their needs for help in terms of their disability. Loss of independence and mobility were among the issues that spouses reported as most problematic. As a result their felt needs for services were likely to be for good quality aids and equipment. Thus, a quarter of spouses, but only one carer (whose partner was not, in any case, fit enough to be interviewed) mentioned a need of this sort. Two spouses felt that they needed or had needed additional community nursing support; one at the time of discharge from hospital (Mr Ord), and one currently to help with her bathing and care during menstruation (Mrs Jefferson).

Two couples (one carer, two spouses) mentioned the need for help with household maintenance tasks; in both cases they were young and buying their own homes. Other interviews also suggested that household maintenance created problems, especially when husbands were disabled:

the heavy jobs around the house. If I didn't have to do those it wouldn't be just so bad . . . Your routine maintenance, trying to keep your house, whereas other couples the husband could do them . . . I think you could do with help. Because I can't do it, we've got to pay someone to do it, and it doesn't come cheap. (Mrs Ord, carer)

As Mrs Ord went on to point out, there was no equivalent of the home help to assist couples when the husband was disabled: 'No, there isn't a man help, is there?'

As might be expected, when their partners relied on them so much for help some carers saw their main service needs in terms of relief or respite from caring or for assistance with child care. Some also felt the need for a break, however temporary, from the sameness of their days:

Interviewer: What sorts of help would you like to see available for people in your sort of position?
[pause] It's nice to get a break sometimes, if that's anything to go by.
Interviewer: Mm, a break for you yourself?
Yeah. Um, something a little bit different. Let somebody else take over for a day or something like that, you know [laugh]. That's all. (Mrs Keighley, carer)

It is difficult to convey with the written word the tentativeness of Mrs Keighley's (and other carers') expression of the wish for some relief from the responsibility of caring. It was almost as if they did not dare voice the wish; indeed, as the above quotation suggests, it was only when asked what help they thought should be provided for people in their sort of position that most carers were able to articulate any of their own needs.

Spouses, too, would have been grateful for the chance to get out of the house, for a change of scenery and for a change of companion. As we shall see in Chapter 6, the lack of occupation during the day and of a social life were major contributors to strain in the couples' relationships.

Conclusions

Those local authority services which were provided to couples in the study were mostly directed towards a reduction of disability rather than directly towards the relief of the carer. Thus, aids and adaptations which made it easier for the spouse to wash, bathe, use the toilet, get up and downstairs, and so on made up the bulk of formal help from this source. Such provision could also reduce the carer's involvement, but in no case did it replace it.

No services were provided which relieved carers altogether from the need to help either. Even among male carers, where there has been evidence from previous studies to suggest a greater likelihood of service provision, there was no suggestion that services were intended to replace the carer *as* carer. The only carers to receive the home help service *were* men, but this may have had as much to do with women carers' perceptions of the inappropriateness of domestic help as it had to do with any discriminatory attitudes on the part of service providers. Male carers accepted the home help service in some sense as a replacement for their wives' domestic services; female carers could see no need for such help as long as they were themselves physically able to do domestic work. Rather, female carers would have been grateful for a home maintenance service which relieved them of the heavy physical tasks associated with maintenance of a house and garden.

Undoubtedly both female and male carers of the most severely disabled spouses would have welcomed the opportunity to have a break from providing care. Their ability to express this need was, in some cases however, constrained by anxieties about the quality of substitute care and their perceptions of greater deservingness in others. The latter was a particular feature of female carers' accounts.

The most serious gaps in the provision of services to spouses and carers occurred when they had been in hospital. Hospital staff had often seemed unable to recognize the need to put couples in contact with social workers, even when it must have been clear that there would be major changes in the couples' lives. Both spouses and carers had been left in extremely vulnerable positions and in some cases had become more ill or disabled, as a result of early discharge, than they were when they entered hospital.

Carers had substantial unmet needs for emotional support, especially at the time of disablement or diagnosis, and both carers and spouses needed information about the nature, prognosis and anticipated effects of the spouse's condition. Without key-workers and without proper communication between hospitals and the community it is difficult to see how these needs could have been met. A handful of couples did have or had had someone who had taken on some aspect of the role of a key worker, but this seemed often to be a matter of luck. Long-term visiting of the district nurse or a close relationship with a young or female GP improved the chances of having a professional helper who acted as a source of information and help or as a point of referral.

Despite the fact that many of the respondents had conditions which required continual medication GPs, with one or two notable exceptions, played a very minor role in helping or advising either spouses or carers. This is not an unexpected finding; studies of disability have shown repeatedly that GPs are highly unlikely to become closely involved in the lives of disabled children or adults

(Glendinning 1983; Parker and Hirst 1987). Even when they do, they frequently know less about disability than do their patients (Morris 1989; Lonsdale 1990). The finding is, however, made the more worrying by continuing suggestions that GPs could play a leading role in the provision of care to disabled people in the community.

Although service receipt was at a low level, services were sometimes refused because of the spouse's reluctance to expose his or her needs to others. As suggested in Chapter 1, spouses and carers negotiate the presentation of the spouse's impairment to the outside world in such a way that it can oblige carers (in particular, women) to take on responsibility for personal care that they might be prepared to let lie elsewhere. As a corollary, female spouses seemed more likely to give in and accept services that they would rather not in order to give their husbands a break. At its baldest, men's needs came before women's regardless of who was the disabled person and who the carer.

The economic effect of caring and disability

Introduction

Research has underlined repeatedly the link between disability and poor financial circumstances (Sainsbury 1970; Blaxter 1976; Hyman 1977; Townsend 1979; Martin and White 1988; Thompson 1990). Disabled people are less likely to be in paid work than their peers, but often have additional expenses associated with their impairments and disability. In addition, family members can find their employment and income, and sometimes their expenditure, affected if they take on responsibility for supporting a disabled person (Nissel and Bonnerjea 1982; Baldwin 1985; Matthews and Truscott 1990; McLaughlin 1990; Glendinning 1992). Yet money is one of the most important cornerstones to an independent life, allowing disabled people to direct their own lives and, where they wish to do so, reduce their reliance on family members, friends and neighbours (Morris 1989). Financial stringency can either be the 'cause or effect of problems of practical care', but is often 'simply the major problem in its own right' which disabled people encounter (Blaxter 1976: 89).

The links between disability and low levels of income are of two sorts. First, poorer people in general and those who are in manual occupations in particular are more likely to become disabled (Blaxter 1976). This is because they are in occupations which are more likely to lead to injury at work or ill-health through work processes. There is also a clear link between socio-economic status and chronic ill-health. Secondly, disability is associated with poor financial circumstances because disabled people experience both direct and indirect discrimination in the labour market. Loss of employment, reduced career opportunities, lost hours of work, poorer rates of pay associated with disability, coupled with the inability of the benefits system to compensate for these losses, all combine to give disabled people a level of financial resources well below that of their non-disabled peers (Martin and White 1988). Those who help and support disabled people at home also experience such disadvantage. Carers may have to give up work, work fewer hours and give up promotion opportunities because there are no supportive services for the disabled person or because available resources are insufficient to meet the costs of personal care (Nissel and Bonnerjea 1982; Baldwin 1985;

Glendinning 1992). For carers, too, there is no benefit which would replace lost earnings for any but the very lowest paid.

The causal links between disability and low income are reflected in two different types of effects among those who become disabled in adulthood (Sainsbury 1970; Blaxter 1976; Locker 1983). For people who have been in poor financial circumstances before they become disabled, disability adds to what has already been a life of financial struggle, while those who have been better off have to accommodate rapidly to substantially reduced circumstances. The first group are unlikely to have had savings or access to occupational pension schemes which might help to buffer them financially. The second group *may* have such provision, dependent upon the nature of the work they did and the type of employer they worked for, but will find themselves using up resources that they had planned to use at a later stage in their life cycle (Sainsbury 1970; Locker 1983).

Other factors which affect the financial resources to which disabled people have access are the way in which they became disabled and their previous status in the labour market. Those who are disabled during service in the Armed Forces or at work, or who suffer from prescribed conditions known to be caused by the type of work they do, are all entitled to higher rates of state benefits than other disabled people. Furthermore, those who have fulfilled certain contribution conditions while in paid work may claim invalidity benefit. Those who do not fulfil these conditions may claim the severe disablement allowance which is paid at a lower rate. Both these factors discriminate indirectly against disabled women (Morris 1989; Lonsdale 1990).

As well as experiencing lower incomes than their peers, disabled people have higher levels of expenditure, making them doubly disadvantaged financially. Extra expenditure can arise in three different ways (Martin and White 1988; Thompson 1990). First, there are lump sum purchases for substantial items, such as housing adaptations, wheelchairs, and cars, which individuals would not otherwise need. Secondly, there is the regular additional expenditure on special items and services such as continence aids or personal and domestic care services. Thirdly, there is extra expenditure on everyday items and services – such as fuel, laundry costs, mortgages. When the disabled person's own income is insufficient to cover these extra expenses other household members find themselves 'subsidizing' the costs of disability (Hoad *et al.* 1990; McLaughlin 1990; Glendinning 1992).

Younger disabled people who have dependent children seem to be particularly badly off. The disability surveys carried out by the British Office of Population Censuses and Surveys (OPCS) showed that *relative to other sorts of households containing disabled adults* married couples with children had low incomes, second only to lone parents, who were the poorest. However, when the number of earners in the household was taken into account, married couples with children were the poorest when there was no earner, one earner, or two earners. It was only the fact that married couples with children *could* have two earners that made them slightly better off, as a group, than single parents.

The existing literature on disability and caring raises a number of issues specific to the position of younger married couples. The most important of these is that of married women and their paid work. Married women have always been seen as peripheral to the labour market – forming part of the reserve pool of labour – and thus to the state benefit system and to the attentions of those who wish to encourage participation in the labour market (Blaxter 1976; Morris 1989; Lonsdale 1990). Married women's primary roles are still seen as those of home-makers and carers, and there is still the widespread assumption that they are, and should be, supported financially by their husbands. As a result, married women's exclusion from the labour market because of disability or because they are caring has rarely been recognized as a real issue.

This is a complicated area for a number of reasons. Some research on disability suggests that married women do not experience the same degree or type of loss when they leave paid work as do men (Sainsbury 1970; Blaxter 1976). Other work suggests that women can experience 'job loss as acutely as . . . men and few [are] content to settle into the role of housewife' (Locker 1983: 113). Certainly, most of the literature on *caring* shows that women experience substantial effects on their paid work and that this causes considerable disquiet. However, if married women do have to give up paid work they do at least have an alternative role which is acceptable both to the world at large and to officialdom, if not to the women themselves (Sainsbury 1970; Blaxter 1976). This is not the case for most men.

A further complication arises because of married women's existing responsibilities for home-making and child care. These, combined with the additional effort required to live life with a physical impairment or to provide substantial help to a disabled person, may make paid work just too much (Sainsbury 1970; Lewis and Meredith 1988; Morris 1989). This is not to condone the unequal division of responsibilities within many marriages, but merely to recognize that for some women such inequalities exist and interact with disability and with caring.

A second and related issue is that of role change. The literature suggests that men feel the loss of paid work most acutely when their partners take over the role of main earner (Sainsbury 1970; Blaxter 1976). Similarly, men who give up paid work to help their disabled wives may feel the difference between their position and that of their peers more acutely than women in a similar situation. The state has itself reflected these different expectations about men and women in that, until relatively recently, the British social security system treated the husbands of disabled women more stringently than the wives of disabled men. This difference was in relation both to the smaller amount which men could earn before their partner's benefits were affected and to the requirement that they should register for work. As we shall see later, the nature of the labour market for men, especially for those in manual occupations, makes it more difficult for them to combine paid work and caring or to be employed part-time after they become disabled. As a result both disabled men and male carers may be more likely than their female counterparts to experience 'once and for all' effects on their paid work.

No study has yet directed its attention exclusively to the economic situation of younger married couples although such couples are likely to be in a particularly precarious position economically. The study reported here was not designed to cost the economic effects of disability and caring for this group, although paid work, income and expenditure were all covered in our conversations. This generated detailed accounts of the nature, rather than the size, of the economic effects of disability. This chapter examines, in turn, the paid work of the carers and their partners, the perceived effects of disability and caring on incomes and expenditure, and changes in household financial arrangements.

The carers' paid work

At the time of the interviews five of the thirteen female carers had paid employment (all part-time), while five of the eight male carers had paid employment (all full-time). Age effects, life cycle effects, and structural differences in male and female labour market participation all had a part to play in the effect which caring had on carers' paid employment, over and above the nature or degree of the spouse's impairments.

Female carers

Among the women carers aged 40 or above three distinct patterns of labour market participation were evident. First, when attachment to the labour market had always been minimal, for example, when women had had no paid work outside the home since the birth of their children, the husband's disability had little or no effect on labour market participation.

Secondly, there were those women who had been intermittently attached to the labour market since marriage or childbirth: they had a series of part-time jobs which they had fitted in around school hours and school holidays. When their children grew some of these women increased the amount of paid work they did. Later on, some had actually given up paid work because of their *own* ill-health before their husbands needed substantial help. In the other cases, however, paid work had either been given up, or had been chosen because it could be fitted around caring. Carers in this sub-group had sometimes been young enough to think about developing their careers, as their children became less dependent, until their husbands' disability or illness intervened.

Finally, among the women aged 40 and above, there was a sub-group that had been very strongly attached to the labour market; they had usually worked full-time since marriage or had taken on substantial employment commitments when their children were still young. It was among this group that there were the most substantial effects on paid work. Mrs Baker had actually been made redundant before her husband needed a lot of help. However, she felt that she would have taken on another job if her husband had not needed her so much. All the other women in this sub-group had either changed from full-time to part-time work, or had given up paid work altogether, because of the need to look after their husbands.

All the female carers under the age of 40 found that the need to look after their husbands had a substantial effect on their labour market participation.

In some cases part-time work was essential to the household's finances but had to be fitted in around the demands of caring:

> before I go to work in the morning I make him a flask, make sure his bottle is within reach. The telephone is always there, his paper, whatever else he needs, make sure he's been to the toilet before I go out to work . . . get him back and he should be all right then until I come home. I work actually a seven minute walk from home, I'm out for three hours. (Mrs Ord, carer)

For women with young children the effect of their need to help their husbands had two distinct phases. First, there was the time when their children were very young when, other things being equal, they might have chosen not to take paid work. However, because of the loss or reduction of their husbands' income they felt obliged to find a paid job, and carried the combined responsibilities of paid work, housework, child care and caring. Sainsbury (1970) discovered a similar pattern among younger carers in her study and there is evidence of a similar effect in the OPCS disablement survey (Martin and White 1988). Secondly, when their children were less dependent, they might have chosen to widen their horizons, take full-time work instead of part-time, or retrain. However, the demands of caring made these prospects unlikely: 'if I could have gone back to work full-time or gone on to do something different [pause] but I don't see me doing anything like that now' (Mrs Ord, carer).

Like Mrs Alston, who had also been under 40 when her husband became disabled, Mrs Ord's ability to participate in the labour market was affected not only immediately, but also, and perhaps more substantially, in the long term. This type of longer term effect is also evident among other groups of women carers, particularly the mothers of disabled children (Baldwin 1985; Glendinning 1985).

Male carers

Age and life-cycle effects were not as obvious or as dramatic among the male carers and all were or had been the principal wage earner in their household. As would be expected, their relationship to the labour market was significantly different from that of the female carers. Although the women being cared for by their husbands had less severe impairments, overall, than the men being cared for by their wives, none of the male carers' paid work had been totally unaffected.

Mr Jefferson gave up work directly because of having to help his wife, but his work had been seriously affected for some three or four years previously. Another husband, Mr Verwood, had actually been dismissed from his job for misconduct, but felt that he would not now be able to return to work anyway because of his wife's condition. Mr Eden was not at work when interviewed, but did have a job to return to. He had been away from work for 18 months because of his own ill-health, but felt that a return to work would be difficult because of his need to help Mrs Eden. He had also lost days at work due to his wife's ill-health before he became ill himself.

Other husbands altered or adapted their pattern of paid work to fit around their caring responsibilities and lost occasional days at work when their wives were ill.

Adapting patterns of paid work

A good proportion of female carers and all the male carers had adapted their pattern of paid work to accommodate the need to help their spouses. The extent of the adaptation required was influenced, obviously, by a combination of the carer's level of participation in the labour market at the onset of the partner's need for help and the level of help required. The combination of full- or part-time work, the onset of the need for a high level of help and the lack of supportive services caused carers to give up work, regardless of their sex:

> we got to the stage where [wife] was falling down a lot and I would be called from work . . . And it came to a head one day when I was called back from work and [wife]

had fallen on the floor, she was trying to get to the toilet, hadn't made it, and her Mum couldn't lift her up . . . and . . . the boys had come in from school and they were crying, [wife] was crying, her Mum was crying and she just said, 'We'll have to do something about it . . .'

We were left, when I did give up work, we were left with the choice of, well no choice really, except that if I hadn't given up work [wife] would have had to go into care. (Mr Jefferson, carer)

he seemed to be doing all right and then this accident occurred so then we decided to, both of us . . . well he couldn't go to work, and I was needed at home. (Mrs Keighley, carer)

When the carers were less intensively involved, paid work could be fitted around or adapted to their responsibilities, but the ways in which this was or could be done varied between female and male carers.

Women were more likely to reduce their hours, take up part-time work when in other circumstances they would have worked full-time, or stay in part-time work for longer than they would otherwise have done.

Mrs Ibstock returned to work after her husband's condition improved temporarily, but she moved from full-time occupation at a factory some distance away to part-time work at a nearby school:

I'm a cleaner over there, the hours . . . is half past six in the morning but you're finished at nine so that's dead handy. I mean, we've got a telephone upstairs in the bedroom and if he ever wakes up and I'm still at work, all he's got to do is lift the phone and phone the school and I'm straight over. Where, if I had any other kind of job, if it was any distance away, it sort of wouldn't work out, you know . . . that's the only reason why I am over there is because it's handy . . . but we've got like an understanding over there, if the phone ever rings and he's not well I just come straight out, so it's handy.

As Mrs Ibstock's experience suggests, work had not only to be part-time, but also nearby to be feasible. Moreover, employers had to be understanding, although this 'understanding' was sometimes bought at a cost to the carer:

You see my gaffer over there he knows I'm a good worker and he knows I never ever stay off unless it's really necessary and I think that's why he's so understanding . . .

I think if the circumstances had been different and I had the flu I would stay off. I mean if he was all right and I had the flu I would just stay off. But I don't know when I'm going to be off because I don't know when these attacks [MS] are going to come. (Mrs Ibstock, carer)

For men whose wives had intermittent needs for a high level of help or who were not so disabled that their husbands had to give up work altogether, the options were a negotiated sick role for themselves, occasional days off work or a different pattern of full-time work.

Men were more likely than women to have experienced unhelpful attitudes from their employers about their need to take time off from work, although this was not a universal experience. However, it was acknowledged that a sympathetic attitude could be expected to extend only so far: '. . . I mean they'll only put up with so much. I mean if it happened [having days off] over and over and over again they're going to get a bit tired having to cover for me aren't they?' (Mr Picton, carer).

Some men had found jobs which offered them more flexibility. Mr Quincy, for example, who supervised a team of industrial cleaners said:

> I please meself what to do and I organise the men accordingly so sometimes I'm
> home, I can be home in the afternoon, I can be home for lunch, I can have a good
> two to two and a half hours at home, you know, which is useful. I can see how things
> are going for the day. If she's not so good and I don't have a lot on that day I can just
> ring in and say, look, I won't be in for the rest of the afternoon – I'll see you
> tomorrow. There's no pressure. That's because we have a good working relationship
> as well . . . It's not everybody can do that, you know, every employer won't do that
> . . . (Mr Quincy, carer)

The weaker link to the labour market which many women have is, of course, one of the major factors which predisposes them to become carers in a variety of situations. Women earn less, they are more likely to be in part-time work, they have responsibilities for the care of children and so on (Martin and Roberts 1984) – all factors which contribute to their often being the 'line of least resistance' when decisions are being made about who becomes the carer for a child or older parents within a family or household (Qureshi and Simons 1987; Ungerson 1987). Within marriage, however, in the absence of support services for the disabled spouse, there really is little option about who becomes the carer. Consequently these factors are apparently of less importance. Indeed, paradoxically, the weaker structural position of women in such situations appears to enhance the options open to them. Because married women are 'expected' to care and, therefore, to work part-time and change jobs often they appear to be able to combine paid work and caring for a spouse more easily. Because married men are not 'expected' to care, are expected to work full-time, and to hold down a steady job, when caring for a wife they appear to be less easily able to combine work and caring responsibilities.

The importance of paid work to carers

Those carers who were in paid work at the time they were interviewed or who had been in paid work and left it because of their spouse's disability, had definite views on its importance. Interestingly, women carers were much more ready or able to articulate their views on this. This could, perhaps, be due to the fact that a higher proportion of the women had actually experienced substantial changes in their pattern of paid work and, therefore, could more easily see what they had lost or gained as a result.

Money was one of the most important aspects of paid work for female carers. In households where finances were not too tightly stretched it meant access to money that was the carers' to do with as they pleased, while in households where money was in short supply any extra the carer could bring in was vitally important.

The opportunity to leave the house and get a break, and the contact with other people were also important:

> it gives me a break when I go over there, I forget all about here and I'm with me mates
> over there and we have a laugh. It's hard work but I mean we have a laugh and that
> takes my mind off [things] and then soon as I put the key back in the front door I've

got to live with it again, and I think if I didn't have my job to go to, I would just go crackers. (Mrs Ibstock, carer)

When the carer was out of the house, for however short a period, it also meant that the spouse was encouraged to retain his or her independence:

if I didn't have a job that took me out of the house [husband] could be more demanding. He could say, 'I want a cup of tea', 'I want a sandwich' or 'Sit me up, I don't feel quite comfortable'. But when he knows I have to go out to do something else then it makes him do more things for himself. (Mrs Alston, carer)

Although paid work outside the home was generally seen in a positive light it inevitably imposed burdens. The younger carers with dependent children, particularly, found the combination of paid work, helping their partners, housework and child care exhausting, and it left them with very little time for themselves.

Carers also carried anxieties about their spouses with them into the work-place: 'I've got half me mind thinking about how he is here, but as long as I know he's on floor and he's not going to move I can cope with that' (Mrs Gifford, carer).

Given that there were substantial advantages to be gained from paid work for carers, not least of which was their own mental health, policies which explicitly or implicitly depend on carers staying at home are likely to be counterproductive. Some carers *had* given up work because they had had no option and financial recognition of this situation could be of value to them. However, they would have preferred options which allowed them to continue in paid work without having to worry about their spouse's care all the time they were out of the house.

Carers who had been relatively young when their spouses had become disabled had often given up hopes of improved careers, growing businesses or, at the very least, a move from part-time to full-time work. Thus, the impact of caring on their labour market participation would be life-long. For some women carers, particularly, with little or no access to occupational pension rights, the prospect of a late middle-age and old age with no husband and little money loomed very large.

The spouse's paid work

At the time of the interviews only one male spouse had paid work. However, he was receiving sickness benefit and after a history of increasing periods away from work was to be redeployed by his employer after assessment and retraining at an employment rehabilitation centre. Six of the eight female spouses were not in paid work and two, who were among the least disabled, had part-time jobs.

Male spouses

The majority of husbands had been finished from their jobs because of their disability or illness, two had been made redundant and had either become ill later or had been unable to find other work, and one was to be redeployed. All had histories of strong attachment to the labour market and some had had only one or two employers during a working life of 20 years or more. The majority had been relatively young men when they had finished work; two had been under 40 and five between the ages of 41 and 50. Only one had been within 10 years of pensionable age when his working life ended.

The relationship between the cause of the spouse's impairment and its impact on their paid work was not as obvious as might have been expected. Even when there had been a sudden injury there had been a period during which these men had clung to the hope of being able to return to work. Two years after his accident and still wearing a surgical corset, Mr Keighley was shocked to be brought before a medical panel and effectively retired. Others, like Mr Gifford, had returned to work, but may have caused themselves further damage: 'I only managed a day [back at work] and I had to ring [the doctor] up straight away . . . he had to give me a couple of weeks for it just to simmer down a bit . . .'.

Men whose condition was deteriorating had also gone on working past the time when their doctors had advised them to give up, even when it was clear that the job was responsible for their condition. Mr Baker, for example, worked in a steelworks, lifting heavy plates of steel all day. Many of his fellow workmen had developed arthritis, as he had, but had moved to lighter jobs. He was reluctant to do so: 'I loved my job and I wanted my job'.

Mr Ibstock had been advised to leave work in 1973 when he had his first attack of multiple sclerosis. Although he did a very heavy job, had several flare-ups and his overall condition was deteriorating, he remained at work until 1983:

> in the yards we had a great big power hammer, you know, it would just come down, squeeze at five ton, and when it came down full-drop . . . it would hit [at] twenty ton. You're talking about maybe one-and-a-half hundredweight of hot steel on a pair of tongs, you turn it over between the hammer coming up and down, you know, somebody would have got killed. It was just too dangerous to do it, so I just told them, you better finish us like, because I wouldn't have been able to keep going . . .

Just over half of these men had either been injured at work or had done a type of work which led to their disability. Another man strongly suspected that his cancer was associated with the dirty atmosphere he had worked in for so many years, but had no medical evidence to support his argument. Only two had received any form of compensation (and only after very long legal battles) and another had a compensation claim still pending some five years after his accident. Similarly, only three received industrial disablement benefit (see below).

Female spouses

Of the six female spouses not in paid work at the time of the interviews four had given up because of their disability or illness. The fifth had given up work when she had a child and had not yet considered returning, and the other had never had paid work. Neither of the two who were in part-time paid work had been in the labour market since getting married.

Of those who had left the labour market two had been quite strongly attached to it. Mrs Newham had been a lone parent for many years before remarrying and had worked full-time until forced to give up, and Mrs Picton had worked full-time until her first child was born, 18 months before being interviewed. The other three had all given up work when they had their children, but returned to part-time work while the children were still quite young.

As with the male spouses, some of these women had struggled on with their jobs even though their impairments were worsening. The women who had recently taken up paid work had both been restricted in the past by their disabilities (and in one case by her husband's attitude). Both had experienced some improvement in their condition and had decided to risk taking jobs outside the home.

The third woman who had not had paid work since marriage would, for religious reasons, have been unlikely to have considered it, even had she been fit enough.

The importance of paid work to spouses

Because so few of the spouses were actually in employment when interviewed, the nature and quality of their accounts of the importance of paid work were inevitably different from those of the carers. Also, because men's relationship to the labour market is different from women's, and because the majority of the spouses were men, the descriptions given were much more concerned with the spouse's identity as a worker and the threat to this that disability had posed. This was particularly the case with men who had worked for many years in the same job:

> I would give everything if I could go back to work now, if a little fairy came and said, 'Jeff, give me everything and I'll put you right and you can go back to work', I'd give everything I had, anything they could have, if I could go back to work. (Mr Ibstock, spouse)

For men who were younger when they came out of work the loss of their role as the main earner, and the money that went with it, seemed uppermost. Being younger also meant that spouses looked ahead to many years without paid occupation:

> I'm quite young at the moment, that's the only trouble, that's the problem. If I was a bit older it wouldn't have made that much difference but with me being a bit younger you see I've got another . . . thirty years work left, which is a lot. If I was 50 odd now, you'd say, well, early retirement and as the climate is now there's no jobs about. (Mr Mead, spouse)

As well as losing a sense of purpose many men, particularly, lost their friends when they came out of work; several spoke with passion of the sense of belonging which contact with mates at work gave them. As Mr Ibstock pointed out, he had often spent more of his waking hours with his workmates than he had with his wife. None of the men who spoke warmly about their friends at work had maintained much, if any, contact with them after. This may have something to do with the context-specific nature of male working class friendship which means that even 'important informal relationships tend to be restricted to the contexts in which they first arose with little effort being made to enlarge them or alter their character by incorporating them into other activities' (Allan 1985: 72).

By contrast, female spouses spoke most feelingly about the loss of independence, especially financial independence, which came with the end of paid work:

> I miss that bit of independence, that you think you're contributing to the household by bringing a wage home . . . I had that independence that whatever we

bought for the home was *ours*, not just his money coming into it, it was ours. I miss that and for ages and ages I hated asking [husband] for money . . . (Mrs Picton, spouse)

Rehabilitation and retraining

The Department of Employment (DE) has a range of schemes and provision for disabled people including financial assistance for adapting the workplace, providing work-related aids and equipment, introducing disabled job-seekers to new employers, rehabilitation and retraining. The DE also has disablement resettlement officers (DROs) who are available at local job centres to help disabled people think about their employment possibilities and direct them to relevant sources of help. Given that over half of the spouses were under the age of 50 when they became unable to continue with their original employment one might have expected that some help of this sort would have been evident.

There was, in fact, very little evidence of this type of help. One spouse, Mr Gifford, was being redeployed by his employer and was due to start attending a rehabilitation centre for assessment. He had also been receiving regular visits from an occupational health nurse who had been talking to him about his future. Only one spouse specifically mentioned having seen a DRO, but had been told that he was 'too disabled' to be helped in any way:

they've had me for medicals and they just won't accept me, they won't try and do anything with me.
Interviewer: Do you feel they've given up on you then?
Well, I don't think it's a feeling, I think it's a fact . . . (Mr Ord, spouse)

Mr Ord himself had come to believe that he was too disabled to take paid work, yet he was a skilled man whose most recent job had been as an office administrator in a voluntary organization. Pain often affected his ability to concentrate and although it was unlikely that he could manage a nine to five job there might have been some scope for flexible, home-based work. Nothing of this sort had ever been suggested, however.

One other spouse, Mr Hazleton, said that he had been called into an office when he had first had the accident which damaged his back, but 'all they could offer me was like watchmaking or something like that'. He had spent all his life working out of doors and felt strongly that he could not settle to a job indoors. He had returned to work as a gardener for another five years, despite continued back pain.

Having been used to working outside was a strong tie for several of the men interviewed. Mr Gifford, although resigned to the loss of outdoors work, was clearly not looking forward to the alternative and Mr Mead, like Mr Hazleton, was very reluctant to contemplate such a radical change:

what they might plan in the future is me sitting down doing something, because there's no way I can go back on the building, digging and doing roofs.
Interviewer: How does that sound to you . . . ?
No, I couldn't do it, I couldn't stay inside and do anything like that, I'm used to the outside all the time.

Some spouses were too seriously impaired (and ill) to contemplate returning to paid work, but there were others for whom lack of day-time activity was a major problem. Most had been involved in heavy industry or heavy outdoor work and they identified strongly with the type of work they had always done. Such rehabilitation as was on offer to these men was unlikely to be welcome or appropriate without substantial preparation beforehand.

Income

One of the most striking things about the incomes of the couples in the study was their variety, both in size and source. Table 5.1 summarizes the normal sources of income from wages and benefits for male and female carers and spouses. In addition half the couples received housing benefit (for rent, rates or both) ranging from £30 per annum to £25 per week.

Although couples were not asked specifically about the size of their incomes, some volunteered the information and for others it was sometimes possible to calculate size of income from the information they gave about its sources. The range of incomes for which information was available ran, in 1988, for couples without dependent children, from £68.55 invalidity benefit plus a certain amount of housing benefit (for rates) to more than £130 per week from invalidity benefit, industrial disablement benefit, reduced earnings allowance, mobility allowance and higher rate attendance allowance – with a rate rebate of £30 per annum and no other housing costs. For couples with dependent children the range was narrower, with incomes from £116.10 per week – made up of the carer's full-time earnings, the spouse's part-time earnings and child benefit – with a rent of £33 per week (two dependent children) to £186.25 – made up of the carer's full-time earnings, severe disablement allowance and child benefit – with a mortgage and no rates rebate (five dependent children).

These figures are given to illustrate the wide variation in household incomes among couples in essentially similar positions. The reasons for the variation were that: male spouses were far more likely than females to be entitled to national insurance benefits and occupational pensions; some male spouses but not others were entitled to occupational pensions, determined, to some extent, by the stage at which they had left paid work; some spouses had access to attendance and mobility allowances; some carers were in paid work; and some spouses had received compensation payments and industrial disablement benefit for injuries sustained at work.

The impact of disability and caring on household income

Both spouses and carers were asked, in their separate interviews, about the ways in which they felt their household income had been affected. This information paints a vivid picture of the financial constraints with which the study households lived.

When it was many years since the spouse had become disabled it was often difficult for couples to look back and see how things were now different. Apart from anything else, many other things might have happened in the intervening

With this body

Table 5.1 Normal sources of income for male and female carers and spouses

Sources of income			
Carers		Spouses	
Female (n = 13)		*Male (n = 13)*	
Part-time earnings	5	Invalidity benefit	12
Child benefit	4	Disablement benefit/reduced earnings allowance	3
Disablement benefit	1		
Retirement pension	1	Occupational pension	6
None	4	Mobility allowance	6
		Attendance allowance (higher rate)	3
		Interest on savings/investments	2
		Statutory sick pay/sickness benefit/full-time earnings	2
*Male (n = 7)**		*Female (n = 7)**	
Full-time earnings	5	Severe disablement allowance	3
Invalid care allowance	1	Child benefit	3
Invalidity benefit	1	Part-time earnings	2
Interest on savings/investments	1	Invalidity benefit	1
		Mobility allowance	1
		Attendance allowance (higher rate)	1

*Data for one couple not analysed.

years which also affected household finances – children being born or leaving home, moving house, changing from being a tenant to being an owner occupier and so on. Among these other events changes in the level of household income which were a direct result of disability might be difficult to disentangle.

Furthermore, effects on household income could be *continuing*. Once-and-for-all change did occur – when people left paid work, for example – but these changes continued to affect household finances over a long period and could be compounded as time passed. Conversely, financial circumstances could occasionally improve over time, for example, when a compensation claim was won or when entitlement to some additional benefit was recognized. Some couples also experienced considerable variation in their household income over time as the spouse moved between full-time earnings, sick pay and back again, or as the carer took days off work or worked shorter hours in order to care. It is unlikely, then, that the effects of disability on household income are either simple or constant.

Experiencing a loss of income

Most couples had experienced a substantial drop in their household income since the spouse had been disabled. A few said that they lost money intermittently, usually due to the male carers' having to take days off work to care, or felt that there had been little change because they had not been very prosperous anyway before the onset of the spouse's disability. Only one couple said that the onset of disability, as such, had made no difference to their household income because the spouse had left work to have a child rather than because of her health problems.

Couples who had experienced both the loss of the main earner's paid work and the loss or reduction of the other partner's income were, not surprisingly, most likely to point to a dramatic drop in their household income, regardless of who was the disabled partner.

For some couples the effect of the spouse's disability was like an imposed early retirement with all that that implied for a reduced income over the long term and the gradual erosion of savings. This was particularly difficult for couples whose income had dropped at just the time when they might have expected to enjoy a little prosperity:

> the point is we should be enjoying ourselves now but there's neither the money or I'm not well enough to enjoy it . . .
> *Interviewer: Because you'd have a bit of money and you'd have a bit of time if you weren't . . .*
> Well . . . the main point is since 1970 when money was big and started to improve, you haven't been earning any, so what you've saved is what you've saved before . . .
> (Mrs Eden, spouse)

Some couples had spent many years living on invalidity benefit and little else, and before that had low incomes from the spouse's and/or carer's work. These couples found it difficult to point to any dramatic change in their financial position. However, the length of time that had elapsed, and the other events that had occurred since the spouse had become disabled, seemed likely to account for at least part of this apparent lack of effect; these couples had been held in the relative poverty of an early stage of a manual worker's life cycle (O'Higgins *et al.* 1988):

> We've never had a lot of money because [husband]'s been off work a long while and he never did have a big wage and with three young ones to bring up. So we've never had a lot of money . . . (Mrs Clifton, carer)

It was this type of couple who had to do the most obvious 'scrimping and scraping'. They talked about economizing on food and fuel, and not being able to afford new clothes, and were clearly less well supplied with consumer goods than were other couples. Moreover, they had little better to look forward to. The male spouses had left paid work too early to benefit from the state earnings-related pension scheme and had no occupational pensions. The only hope – if such is the word to describe it – they had of their household income increasing was if the spouse's condition deteriorated and he or she became eligible for mobility or attendance allowance.

Some households experienced fluctuations in their income which made forward planning particularly difficult:

he seemed to have intermittent periods, because he'd start back and think everything would be all right and it would get too rough or too difficult. And then he'd have another month off and then he'd work maybe a fortnight and have another month off. And it went sort of intermittent and you never really got the chance to build anything up financially. (Mrs Alston, carer)

Expenditure

As outlined at the beginning of this chapter, disability and poor financial circumstances can be related both to reduced income and increased expenditure. Questions about changed patterns of expenditure obviously touched on important issues for couples and triggered a large amount of detail. This is presented here in two sections: one which covers the major goods or services on which more or less was being spent; and one which covers more general issues about changes in household budgeting practices.

Expenditure on goods and services

Fuel
Most couples felt that they spent more on fuel to heat their homes than they would otherwise have done. There were two main reasons given for this: the need to heat the house throughout the day when, in the past, it would have been empty; and the spouse's need for a warmer environment than normal.

Mr Ord spoke about his extra expenditure on fuel in terms of the lengths to which he had to stretch his income:

> It's not only the income, it's the income in relation to the expenditure, because also at this stage, I wouldn't be expecting to heat the house 24 hours a day, virtually. I would have expected to be out working so I would have had lower overheads. I mean our fuel overheads for this house, as small as it is, are tremendous, and I think that we are fairly frugal. (Mr Ord, spouse)

Extra heating was not the only reason for additional fuel expenditure. When Mrs Fowey's husband developed colitis she did far more washing of clothes and bedding than usual, and noticed a substantial increase in her electricity bill the following quarter.

It was not necessarily how disabled a spouse was which had an effect on household fuel use, but rather his or her presence in the house throughout the day. The effect of the disability was, rather, to make it more necessary that heating should be kept on, because it was difficult for the more disabled spouses to keep warm, often because of circulation problems or impaired mobility.

Transport
Expenditure on transport had changed for different couples in different ways. First, there were those couples who reported that they *had* to run a car when, perhaps, they might not otherwise have done, and secondly, there were those who said that they had given up running a car or could not afford to do so because their income was too low.

Interestingly, the first group – those who said they had to run a car – did not include all the spouses whose mobility was most impaired nor, by implication, all those who received mobility allowance (MA).

Although some spouses might not be sufficiently immobile to qualify for MA they still needed to be transported in a car because their impairment made the use of public transport difficult. Mrs Eden, for example, could walk, but could get only a short distance before she was 'caught short'. When in the car she stayed drier for longer and felt much more at ease. Similarly, Mr Rutland could walk, but became very breathless when he went more than a hundred yards or so, especially when the weather was windy.

Some couples (one of whom received MA) had given up running a car because they could not afford it. In three of these cases the wives had been learning to drive, but had given up having lessons either because they were too expensive or there seemed little point when there was no longer a car. In all these cases the wives were learning because their husbands had become unable, or might become unable, to drive as a result of their disability. This course of action had, however, been cut short by a lack of money. These couples then became dependent on public transport, which the spouse could often not use, or taxis.

The receipt of MA appeared to enable couples who already had a car to keep it running after the spouse had become disabled although the cost of petrol and maintenance (if not using the Motability scheme) still created problems. However, when the spouse was severely disabled – and thus had other additional expenses – *and* had other mobility needs, such as a wheelchair, MA was not sufficient to enable the couple to continue running a car.

Food

As with transport, couples talked about spending less on food generally because there was less money available or spending more because the spouse had special dietary requirements. In fact, both effects were sometimes evident in the same household.

Mrs Derby's account of the time when her husband was gravely ill and she was trying to build him up illustrates vividly the relationship between money devoted to one element of household expenditure and that available for other elements:

> It was an expensive time in regards to, I had to buy – well I felt I had to buy, sort of build him up, he were so thin – like Complan, Build-up, fruit, all extras like that, and they are expensive. But I did feel that I had to do this 'cos if he hadn't have had good food, good nourishment, he'd never have got over this, no way.
> *Interviewer: And did you go without in order to provide what you felt he needed?*
> Well, not really, no [hesitates].
>   Well I cut down. I suppose I did cut down in all sorts of things really. I cut down in everything I use, household things – soap powder, polish, I go without polish and it sounds silly that, but it costs a lot. So these are things that you can really manage without, although they're luxuries really aren't they when you've not much money.

Although the interviewer did not press Mrs Derby, her hesitation over whether or not she had cut back on her own food (either quantity or quality) gave the strong impression that she had.

It is not surprising that it was female carers who were most likely to mention that they had made economies on food expenditure, although some spouses had wondered how their partners had managed financially, especially when they (the spouse) had been particularly ill.

For those households who had always been on a relatively low income it was difficult to recognize any reductions; rather they had always been careful:

> Usually for us the limit is about £40 a week for food but that ends up paying the milk bill and that, you know, and bits and pieces too, so we don't have enough to spend a lot with. We could do with eating a bit better I must admit but it's just not possible at the moment. (Mr Quincy, carer, two adults and two children in household.)

The economies that *were* made, when money was in short supply, were on the quality of food bought:

> We can't buy what we would really like to buy at times – I have to go for the cheaper cuts. Things like that. Now on a Sunday, sometimes I'll buy a small joint, and sometimes I won't. I'll say, no, I'll do a steak and kidney, or mincemeat. Something like that. (Mrs Baker, carer)

All the economizing, both on food and other goods, added another element to the carer's responsibilities, discussed in more detail in the later section on household budgeting.

Household maintenance and decoration

Half the couples mentioned that they now had to pay more for household maintenance or decorating than they had previously. This was usually because male spouses had been able to do these tasks in the past, but could no longer. In several households female carers had taken on responsibility for some of these jobs, but the rest were beyond their physical capabilities. As would be expected, this was especially the case for the older women.

One factor which influenced whether or not couples had to pay for household maintenance was tenure. Couples who had bought their council house or who had moved from local authority accommodation into owner occupation no longer benefited from local authority help with maintenance. The Giffords, for example, needed their house repointing and a new fence erecting. Mrs Gifford could do so much, but not all of either task; consequently they would have to pay someone else to do the work. When the carer could not do the job and money was in short supply quite important tasks went undone:

> We had a leak [in the roof] – see he used to be able to do all that himself, now we have to get people in and we can't at the moment because we can't afford it . . . Most of the things now he just has to leave them, but we will eventually have to get someone in, with moving [and selling the house]. (Mrs Mead, carer)

We can see here, again, that disability can increase household expenditure but that, when income is inadequate, it can also cause expenditure to be reduced or delayed even on quite important items or services.

Clothes and shoes

Expenditure on clothing and shoes was affected in exactly the same way as the other goods and services discussed so far. Some couples, especially those on the lowest incomes, said that they could not easily afford new clothes and shoes while others described how they had to spend *more* on the disabled spouse's clothes and shoes because of special needs.

Some spouses had had substantial losses or gains of weight and had to have new clothing. Others wore through clothes and shoes more quickly or needed extra clothes because they had to change them frequently:

> The clothing has to be washed more, it gets an accident or whatever, it gets wet, gets something spilt on it much more than you would normally so it gets washed a lot more. So she has to have quite a few changes. (Mr Jefferson, carer)

> at one time he used to slur one of his legs, slur one of his feet and he used to go through shoes. One shoe I used to have at the repairer's about once a fortnight. (Mrs Clifton, carer)

Male spouses and carers seemed particularly upset about the fact that it was difficult to afford new clothes or shoes, perhaps because it was closely tied up with their image of themselves as good providers and husbands:

> it [marriage] would be a lot happier if we were financially better off I think. We don't dwell on it but there are things I know Janet'd like, there's things I'd like you know, such as new clothes. I mean I know she'd like new shoes for one thing, I know she'd like new undergarments but as things are at the present we've got to get the bills out of the way first . . . (Mr Derby, spouse)

Prescriptions

Most of the spouses in the study had medication costs, most were in receipt of benefits of one sort or another, but few had automatic entitlement to free prescriptions. Some had eventually negotiated free prescriptions after long periods of paying out substantial sums for medication, while others were still paying for their drugs.

The interviews revealed substantial confusion about entitlement to free prescriptions even among people who had automatic rights to them because they had a specified condition such as diabetes. This confusion was most evident in relation to the mobility criterion which makes prescriptions free of charge for people who have a physical disability which prevents them from leaving their home except with the help of another person. Confusion was confounded in some cases by the dual channels of DHSS (as it then was) and Family Practitioner Committee (FPC) – now the Family Health Services Authority – through which exemption could be obtained. Professionals were often as ignorant about entitlement, which made it even more difficult for people to fight their way through the system:

> I was paying for my own prescriptions 'till last year and I've been off [work] over six year. And I said to the doctor, 'Do you think that's right that I should be paying, I've been off work a long time'. He said, 'Well get a yearly certificate which is cheaper', which I did. And then I had another go at him. I said, 'Look, I'm saving money but I'm still spending money, and I've paid money into this society, and I'm still having to pay. They're taking my sick money back off me'. He said, 'Well, it's only £30 odd a year'. 'Well £30 odd is a lot of money to me now'. . . He just laughed it off. But when the other doctor came after I came out of hospital . . . I said, 'Do you think it's right that I should pay for my prescriptions, Dr . . .' Well, he said, 'I don't know but, look I'm not going to interfere with it. Tell your wife to go down to DHSS and get this

form thing'. And she went and got it . . . And she went and got the form and I filled it
in and she took it to the doctors. And now I don't pay. So I've saved that money. (Mr
Baker, spouse)

Mr Baker's experience was not atypical. Even Mr Hazleton, who was diabetic
and who, therefore, should have received free prescriptions automatically, had
paid for his prescriptions for several years before a chance remark made by the GP
to his wife revealed that he was eligible for help.

When prescriptions were not free and even when a 'season ticket' had been
bought, the cost of medication made a significant impact on a couple's household budget. If the carer was also unwell his or her prescription charges could
strain the household finances further. Because exemption on the grounds of a
specified condition (rather than because of low income) applied only to the
spouse, carers were still having to pay for their own medication:

I get my prescriptions free of charge. I have Family Practitioner's Committee exemption certificate. I think the grounds that I've got it on is because I am unable to go out
by myself.
Interviewer: But you don't get free prescriptions for your wife and son?
Well for my son I do because he's not 16, but my wife doesn't. (Mr Ord, spouse, wife
suffers from colitis and is on permanent medication.)

Additional expenditure on medication could also extend beyond prescribed
drugs. Mrs Ibstock, for example, bought her husband, who had MS, sunflower oil
capsules:

it costs me £48 for them. We don't get them free, £48, he gets them every six months.
They're supposed to sort of build the myelin up in the spine but they don't – that
hasn't been proved yet at the [hospital] so, what they don't believe in you can't
claim.

Obviously, for as long as Mr Ibstock *felt* the capsules were helping him Mrs
Ibstock wanted to go on buying them.

Leisure activities
One of the areas in which many of the couples mentioned reducing their expenditure was their leisure activities, either through a reduced social life or no longer
taking holidays. It was sometimes difficult to disentangle enforced reductions in
spending on a social life because of the spouse's disability from those due to a lack
of money: 'We used to always go out of a weekend but we don't now so I mean I
save money there, well, if you can call it saving. I never go out and he just can't go
out' (Mrs Ibstock, carer). In other cases the relationship was less equivocal:

I think [husband]'s as browned off as I am, he's not a person who likes to be kept in.
'Course money's not plentiful, I mean there isn't the money to do what he'd like to
do and, of course, there's no holiday. (Mrs Eden, spouse)

As Mrs Eden's comment suggests a reduced social life had more than just
financial implications. Not being able to get out as often as before, and particularly not being able to take a holiday, put a substantial strain on some couples. The importance of getting a break and getting away will be discussed in
more detail in following chapters.

Aids and adaptations

Over half the couples had bought aids to daily living or paid for services or adaptations to their homes which they might otherwise have been able to obtain free of charge from the local authority or health service (see Chapter 4). In addition one couple was making a financial contribution towards a day centre service and another couple was meeting part of the cost of further adaptations to their home.

The range of expenditure was from a few pounds for items such as urine bottles or bath handles, through £100 or more for the installation of a shower, to some thousands of pounds for house adaptations.

Household budgeting

One major financial consequence of the spouse's disability was that couples had to be more careful with household finances. As might have been expected, carers and female spouses were most likely to make this sort of comment.

For some couples – the few who were slightly more prosperous – having to be careful might involve cutting down on birthday and Christmas present expenditure, fewer holidays, a restricted social life or less expenditure on home improvements. For the majority of couples, however, and the women in particular, it was a matter of making household income stretch far enough to cover basic expenditure:

> Sometimes the housekeeping money's got to have a bit of elastic on it to make it stretch . . . 'cos I've had to be careful with money . . .
> Every week I pay something, so I've got like me different dates for different things and I pay something every week so that we're not in Queer Street. All right, I mean folks might think, well we haven't much at end of day, but everybody's paid and we get by . . . (Mrs Hazleton, carer)

Making ends meet increased the physical, as well as the psychological responsibilities of some. They talked about doing more labour-intensive cooking of cheap foods instead of using convenience foods and some, especially when they had young children, had knitted and sewn clothes, and had done much making-do and mending.

Occasionally, male spouses were prompted to wonder how their wives managed on the money available but, as some acknowledged, their preoccupation with their own illness and pain made it difficult to be fully aware of the carer's struggles:

> It has been hard on her, I couldn't do nothing to help [financially]. I've got to be honest with you, it didn't even dawn on me to give much thought to it, because I was feeling so sorry for meself, I won't say sorry, I was in so much pain, not knowing what was happening to me . . . It didn't enter me head [to wonder] how [wife] was getting on. (Mr Keighley, spouse)

> When you're ill money's nothing, money don't come into it, 'cos if you're ill you don't care a damn about money, in fact you'd give all money you'd got to be well again. So I suppose it hit [wife] more than me because she'd got to manage, I was just laid there, she'd got to go on managing and worrying . . . (Mr Derby, spouse)

Only one male carer had taken over entire responsibility for household expenditure and budgeting, which he clearly did not enjoy. Overall, then, women did the coping, regardless of whether or not it was they who were disabled.

Using up savings

Many of the couples were at a stage in their lives when they might otherwise have expected to be at their most prosperous. Their children had left home, they were at the age when people usually command their greatest income, and if they had bought a house when young the mortgage payments were small or were coming to an end. They were also at a stage when they might have expected to be thinking forward to their old age by saving and by replacing household goods to see them through retirement.

In fact, these couples were doing the opposite; they had used up, or were in the process of using up, savings, redundancy money or compensation payments to make up for the loss of the spouse's and/or carer's income, and increased expenditure.

Mr and Mrs Baker used his and her redundancy money to replace household goods in the hope that they would last through an unexpectedly protracted retirement. Mrs Selsdon had also spent savings on making life a little easier for herself and her husband:

> I've got a little bit of savings but I doubt if there's £1 a week interest on them. Most of the savings have been spent since he took ill.
>
> I bought him a new bed for down here. I bought him his chair – I thought, well, he doesn't want to sit in a wheelchair all the time – the recliner chair. You know, things like that. 'Fridge-freezer. I just had the 'fridge before with a freezing compartment and when I can't get out so much to get shopping in, I have the freezer and I can keep plenty of stuff in. It doesn't matter if I don't get out . . . Changed me washer, I had a twin-tub, well I got rid of that and got an automatic 'cos at the start I had a lot of washing. (Mrs Selsdon, carer)

Other couples just saw their savings dwindle as they used them to help compensate for substantial reductions in their income:

> he had good money for years and we used to go away on holidays and all that and then it was just stopped and then the money we had in the bank, well that went, that slowly dwindled away. (Mrs Ibstock, carer)

Mr and Mrs Jefferson had seen two substantial capital sums drain away – one from Mr Jefferson's business and the other from the sale of their house – because they could not claim supplementary benefit (now income support) and because Mrs Jefferson's Severe Disablement Allowance and Mr Jefferson's Invalid Care Allowance were not sufficient to live on:

> we had to use up any monies that I'd acquired through me business . . . [I] struggled by for quite a while without realising that I'd come below a level where I was eligible for supplementary benefit . . .
> *Interviewer: . . . and then you sold the house and had to live on that?*
> Yeah . . . we still do in a sense.
> *Interviewer: Because you're still not getting supplementary benefit?*
> Well, no, we don't get supplementary benefit.

For couples who had been young when the spouse became disabled there had simply been no opportunity to build up savings.

The OPCS report on the financial circumstances of disabled adults (Martin and White 1988) has suggested that use of savings by people with disabilities is not an indicator of financial difficulties. The report points out that only people who had previously had high incomes have any savings to use up and that 'many people save for their retirement or for large items of expenditure and expect to use their savings' (p. 70). This is, of course, true. However, the use of savings or windfalls *was* problematic for married couples in this study because they were using them at a much earlier stage in their lives than they would otherwise have done, leaving them potentially vulnerable – and certainly more vulnerable than their peers – as they aged. Younger couples were even more disadvantaged because they would never be able to build up savings for their retirement and had no opportunity to build up additional pension rights. Many of these couples faced the prospect of a financially bleak old age.

Changes in patterns of household financial management

The 'black box' of household financial management and its relationship to power within marriage has recently started to attract the attention of social researchers (Pahl 1980, 1989; Brannen and Wilson 1987; Wilson 1987). The different patterns of responsibility which married couples adopt, and whether and how they change over time have now been examined in some detail. Evidence about whether or not patterns change in response to major life events, such as major illness or disability is, however, scant.

The most striking thing to emerge from this study was the persistence of household financial management strategies despite major life changes. Two-thirds of the couples said that the way in which they sorted their money out had remained essentially unchanged. However, whether or not and how much these patterns could or needed to change was determined to a large extent by what they initially were.

For example, if the partners had previously worked full-time and each had taken responsibility for meeting particular bills [the independent management system in Pahl's (1989) model], either giving up paid work would make re-arrangement essential. By contrast, if a male breadwinner had always 'tipped-up' his wage to his wife and had pocket money only returned to him (the whole wage system) the change from a wage to a benefit would not necessarily make a re-arrangement of responsibility urgent. The sex of the spouse who became disabled and the nature of the disability might also be likely to influence whether or not changes took place.

Nine couples had used the whole wage system with the wife responsible for managing the money before the spouse's disablement and only one of these had changed this pattern subsequently. In this one case the husband had taken over complete responsibility when his wife's condition had deteriorated so much that she was no longer intellectually capable of dealing with money.

Six couples had used an allowance system (where the husband gave his wife a housekeeping allowance each week, but retained money and responsibility for payment of some major bills) before the spouse became ill or disabled, but four had changed subsequently, either to a different system altogether or to a modified version of the allowance system. Mr and Mrs Derby had moved to a whole wage system, Mr and Mrs Eden and Mr and Mrs Ord to a pooled system (where both partners pooled their income and both had access to it), and Mr and Mrs Keighley to a modified allowance system whereby Mrs Keighley knew much more about their joint finances than she had in the past. In this last case responsibility for payment remained the same – Mr Keighley worked out the finances and sent off the money and Mrs Keighley had a housekeeping allowance – but Mrs Keighley actually knew what was going on, which she had not done in the past.

The need for the female carer to know more about what was going on financially also cropped up in discussion with Mrs Ord. Before becoming disabled Mr Ord had dealt with all household financial affairs, apart from housekeeping: 'Now we both do it, so we both know where it's going. But I actually do all the banking and that. I go to the places to pay, but we work the money out between us' (Mrs Ord, carer). Mrs Ord felt much happier about this arrangement because if anything happened to her husband she would know where she was financially.

Mrs Baker did not have this reassurance. The Baker's had previously used an independent management system (one of only two examples of this model in the study):

> Well when she was working she said to me, 'You pay the mortgage and you pay the electric, I'll pay the gas and I'll pay the food'. And she had her bit of money in the bank and I had my bit of money in the bank. (Mr Baker, spouse)

Since they had both stopped work, however, Mr Baker had taken over completely and Mrs Baker had no independent access to any of their money:

> If anything happened to him tomorrow I wouldn't have a clue . . . He does all the paperwork. He sorts all the bills out. He has little piles of money here. The tea lad's coming – that's for the tea lad, that's for the milkman and so on. And that's every week (Mrs Baker, carer).

Mr Alston had also taken over complete responsibility for household finances when he stopped work although Mrs Alston did have a bank account of her own into which half her wages was paid; she was responsible, with the other half, for meeting the telephone bill. In addition, the reduced rent for their house, which was a perk of her job, was stopped directly from her wages.

In all cases where male spouses had taken substantially increased control over household finances carers tended to explain their acceptance of this in terms of giving the spouse something to do. For the spouse the justification for the change was also in terms of relieving their wives of a burden or being able to put money aside for the wives so that they would be protected in the future should anything happen to them (the spouses):

> I handle the money now, to give me something to do. I handle the money. If anything happened to me, [wife] would be all right. But [wife] don't bother with the money now but she did when [I was ill] she used to have to do all the housekeeping. It's just to give me something to do. (Mr Keighley, spouse)

Finally, two couples who had used the pooling system of allocation retained this system after the spouse had become disabled although in one case the spouse had not yet been forced to give up work.

The impact of the spouse's disability on household financial management was complex, then. Contrary to what might have been expected, spouses were more likely to gain control than were carers. When the spouse was physically unable to deal with money and paying bills then the carer might gain *responsibility* for management, but this did not always bring controlling power with it. Furthermore, whether or not changes did take place was influenced by the previous patterns which were, in turn, influenced by the carer's gender and previous relationship to the paid labour market.

Conclusions

This is perhaps the most difficult chapter from which to draw conclusions because as we have seen, the effect of disability on financial circumstances depends so much on what the prior circumstances were and which partner became disabled.

One of the most disturbing things to emerge is the position of households where it is the wife who has become disabled. Because of the lower likelihood of women being entitled to contributory and occupational benefits, such households were significantly worse off than similar households where the husband was disabled. Furthermore, because of the ways in which they became disabled, women were less likely than men to be receiving industrial disablement benefits which are substantially more generous than other disablement benefits.

The traditional patterns of male labour market participation also compound the effects of disability on households containing a disabled woman. Because men are less likely to have access to part-time paid work, and in the absence of adequate support services, they are more likely to have to give up paid work altogether when their wives start to need significant amounts of help.

To say that households with disabled wives in them might be worse off than others is not, however, to suggest that the others were doing well financially. The only couples who were comfortable financially were those who had received compensation payments or who had had substantial capital in the past and generous occupational pension provision at the present. All the other couples where the spouse was significantly impaired had experienced decreases in their incomes, or increases in their expenditure, or both. When the couple were older they experienced the financial effects of retirement 10–15 years earlier than they would otherwise have done. When the couple were younger they saw before them a lifetime of scrimping and scraping with little or no opportunity to save, and no prospect of a relatively prosperous middle age once their children were grown. Disability thus caused major shifts in the expected life cycle pattern of household economics.

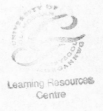

Disability, caring
and marriage

Introduction

Marriage, both 'normal' and dysfunctional, has been the subject of much academic study and thought over the last 25 years (Clark 1991). Researchers have examined the nature of marriage from a variety of sociological and psychological viewpoints: they have argued that it is a 'symmetrical' relationship (Young and Wilmott 1975), they have argued that it is not (Oakley 1974), they have examined it in its early years (Mansfield and Collard 1988), when it is in trouble (Brannen and Collard 1982), and when it has ended (Dominian 1985). In addition, there is a growing literature on marital therapy based, for the most part, on psycho-dynamic theories (e.g. Rogers 1973).

Despite this large (and growing ever larger) literature there is very little information about disability and marriage or family life more generally (Sainsbury 1970; Blaxter 1976; Locker 1983; Morris 1989; Creek *et al.* not dated). The work that *is* available in this field tends to deal with the needs of people with learning disabilities, people who have been physically disabled since birth or childhood (e.g. Craft and Craft 1983), or those who have experienced spinal injuries (Hoad *et al.* 1990).

The literature on disability does contain some references to the experience of married people (e.g. Sainsbury 1970; Blaxter 1976, Locker 1983) and there have been some accounts of spouse carers in the informal care literature (Thompson 1987; Ungerson 1987). This work has suggested a number of issues that are likely to be important for younger couples where one partner becomes disabled after marriage.

The first of these is about roles within the relationship. Despite what might be popularly held about changed roles within marriage, there is little evidence to suggest any major shifts among the majority of couples (Finch and Morgan 1991; Finch and Summerfield 1991; Richards and Elliot 1991). As Finch and Morgan (1991) sum up, the 'clear evidence of research in the 1980s was that men's and women's respective domestic roles, and the gender relations which these embodied, had changed remarkably little' (p. 64). As a result, married men largely see themselves as responsible for the major financial contribution to the marriage while women see themselves as responsible for domestic work and child care (even if they are also earners). As we saw in earlier chapters, disability sometimes means substantial shifts in these conventional responsibilities, with all that this implies for challenges to accepted roles. Some studies have suggested that such challenges put strain on marriages (Sainsbury 1970; Hoad *et al.* 1990). Others have pointed out that it is not so much role reversal which causes difficulties but rather 'role overload' when the partner takes on some or all parts of the disabled person's role (Oliver 1983).

A related issue is that of what partners expect of one another. By and large, married men still expect their wives to provide them with domestic services and some aspects of personal care, while married women do not expect such services from their husbands. If wives take on responsibility for their husband's personal care after the onset of disability, then it may be difficult for the husbands to see what their wives do. Furthermore, some men may not judge the provision of such help as in any way problematic (Sainsbury 1970; Oliver 1983) and may be reluctant to have any one else provide it (Oliver 1983; Hoad *et al.* 1990; and see Chapters 2 and 4). By contrast, if husbands take on responsibility for their wives' personal care or start to provide domestic services, this provision may be only too visible to the wife and cause her feelings of guilt or inadequacy (Sainsbury 1970; Morris 1989). Morris (1989), in summing up the experiences of spinally injured women, says, 'Some of us find that a relationship with a man is under added strain following our disability because our roles as women are so bound up with caring for a male partner. Some men find it very difficult to take on the caring role' (p. 85).

Disability may also change or, alternatively, reinforce existing power differences in relationships. On the one hand, carers may gain control over some aspects of the couple's life together, thus increasing power for the wives of disabled men (particularly over financial matters (Hoad *et al.* 1990) although as we saw in Chapter 5, this is not universal) and decreasing power for disabled women, as their partners take over control in areas which had previously been the women's domain (Morris 1989). On the other hand, carers (particularly women) may lose power if their partner's disability becomes the main focus of their lives together.

The pre-existing quality of the marriage and, indeed, the personalities of the individuals involved may be crucial in understanding what happens to the couple after the onset of disability (Locker 1983; Nichols 1987). Most marriages seem to survive, but whether or not they do is also related to the extent to which the partners are able to *negotiate* adjustment to their changed lives (Locker 1983; Hoad *et al.* 1990; Creek *et al.* not dated). Adjustment is made more difficult, however, by lack of support. In the absence of paid employment or other daytime activity outside the home couples can be thrown together for 24 hours a day; without adequate equipment, adaptations or services carers can buckle under the physical and emotional strain of helping their partners; and providing intimate personal care can mean that the partner/lover becomes the nurse/care attendant with consequent strain on the couple's sexual relationship.

Some marriages *do* break up and this is usually soon after the onset of disability. In some cases the marriage was already rocky; in far more the absence of support and advice forces couples apart (Blaxter 1976; Oliver 1983; Nichols 1987). As Sainsbury observed more than 20 years ago:

it seem[s] ironic that those husbands or wives who had been deserted occupied so much of the time of social workers . . . while none of those for whom the problems were just being created – the newly impaired whose marriages were obviously crack-ing – had been referred for the practical help or emotional support which might have averted the crisis. (Sainsbury 1970: 206)

Other marriages survive; indeed, some couples feel that their experiences have strengthened and enriched the relationship (Sainsbury 1970; Morris 1989; Hoad *et al.* 1990). Others have continued with marriages which were otherwise empty because of a sense of obligation to marriage itself (Oliver 1983; Hoad *et al.* 1990). However, as we shall see in the rest of this chapter, survival is often the result of hard psychological work for both partners.

This chapter is in four main sections. First, we look at the specific aspects of couples' situations which they felt had affected their relationship and marriage. Secondly, the effect of the spouse's impairments on the couple's physical rela-tionship is examined. In the third main section we start to explore both carers' and spouses' views about the nature and meaning of marriage, and how this related to their continuing relationship. Finally, by comparing different mar-riages, and also by comparing the same marriages at different points in time, we attempt to throw some light on what might predispose marriages to break up, after one of the partners becomes disabled.

Pain and bad temper

Pain is, perhaps, one of the most prevalent accompaniments of physical impair-ment (Astin *et al.* 1991), but one of the most difficult to deal with both for those who experience it and those who live with them (Locker 1983; Morris 1989; Hoad *et al.* 1990). People cope with pain often by withdrawing from others both be-cause others do not understand it and because 'the effort of managing pain consume[s] already depleted reserves of energy leaving little to be invested in routine interaction' (Locker 1983: 135).

The negative effect on their relationship which was mentioned most often, both by carers and by spouses, was the spouse's increased bad temper. This was often explained as being due to his or her pain. Spouses with chronic back or joint conditions were particularly likely to be included here although other conditions, such as peripheral vascular disease and advanced multiple sclerosis, also caused pain. Spouses were as aware of their bad temper as were the carers:

We might get on each other's nerves now and again, usually it's my fault, because I usually get a bit, with the condition I have, I get a bit humpty and I get a bit irritable . . . so if there's any fault, if there's any blame to be laid on anybody . . . through us getting on each other's nerves, it should be laid at my door. (Mr Gifford, spouse)

He does get crabby 'cos we're niggly with one another a lot . . . I just think, 'Oh well, he's in pain'. I mean I probably let a lot of things ride because I know what he's going through. (Mrs Gifford, carer)

Frustrations at the limitations imposed by physical impairments also played a part. These outbursts of temper inevitably caused sadness and, in some spouses, a great sense of guilt:

I feel so awful because she's got to wash me and do all she does for me and tend to me and at the end of the day I'm in a lot of pain and I'm not very nice sometimes, I don't want her or nothing. And I feel sorry afterwards, it's nothing to do with her, it's me . . . (Mr Keighley, spouse)

Carers tended to cope with these changes and outbursts by distancing the spouse's behaviour, like Mrs Ibstock who said 'you've just got to let him go on because I know it's not him, you see . . .' , but it hurt nonetheless.

Carers, too, admitted to getting angry, but again, there was the realization that the anger was not real:

occasionally I could just let fly. I let go of me temper sometimes, but I've got to say to [husband], 'Look, just ignore me – pretend I haven't said it, or you haven't heard me get me temper up'. I need to do [it]. You can't just plod on and it not get you without your emotions somewhere. (Mrs Clifton, carer)

Sometimes the bad temper of one partner fed off the bad temper of the other, but they were mostly able to recognize this for what it was: 'things go wrong in the house, you know, and we can't get fixed right away, it's not fair, she must get bad tempered, and I get bad tempered but we know it's all due to the accident, strain and that' (Mr Mead, spouse).

Some carers spoke about how they suppressed their anger because they did not want to upset their spouse:

You've got to put your tongue between your teeth because when he gets to this stage he gets very bad tempered and if things are not done straight away he's liable to explode and you just feel like having a really good row and clearing the air and that's it, but you can't. You've got to put your tongue between your teeth. (Mrs Ibstock, carer)

Others had moved beyond that stage to a less restricted way of interacting: 'Yes, I can shout at him as well, yes. I didn't at first, I didn't think it was right to shout at him, but I do now, yes' (Mrs Ord, carer).

Both carers and spouses were saddened by the increased bad temper in their lives but, for the most part, coped with it by understanding how it arose and distancing themselves from it.

Living on top of one another

Bad temper and irritableness were sometimes associated with the carer and spouse being with one another for much longer hours than was previously the case. Obviously, this was related to loss of paid work outside the home, whether of the spouse or of the carer. Many strongly believed that people were not designed to spend all their time with one another in that way. This was regardless of their sex and of whether they were the carer or the spouse:

It's a strain on us at times, I'll admit, 'cos we're together so much, you do get on each other's nerves, it's only natural. (Mrs Gifford, carer)

I don't know how these old timers retire, you know, they're in each other's pockets all the time. I think it's best to be separated a bit so you can have a bit of time with your own private thoughts. (Mr Ibstock, spouse)

Being together all the time meant there was rarely anything new to talk about and partners became frankly bored with one another:

> we sort of get on each other's nerves because we're together all the time where before he was out all day and I was out all day. He used to come in of a tea-time and he used to tell us what had happened at work and I used to tell him what had happened at work and we always had something to say, where when you're in a house with somebody constant, day after day, night after night, you just lose the sense of conversation, you get to the stage where you don't know what to talk about. (Mrs Ibstock, carer)

Couples who managed to avoid these sorts of feelings were those few who had been able to maintain some social life, often connected with their church, or where either partner was still in paid work.

Some carers felt that their spouses had become very possessive as their physical impairments worsened. This made it even more difficult for these carers to have any time of their own:

> it's very convenient for her, me being there, and she'll say, well get us the ash tray, I'll have a cup of tea, I'll have a drink and so on, and so I do get annoyed [then] I say, well look, I'm going to have an hour on my own and there's still ructions on. There's even ructions on if I go in the bath – 'Why are you going in the bath, make sure that you have your shave, and put your after-shave on' – extreme possessiveness. And I think a lot of it has to do with the fact that I am there all the time . . . (Mr Jefferson, carer)

> he's getting to the stage now where I can't move. If I go upstairs he wants to know where I am and if he had his own way he would get us to pack my job in and just stop in with him all day. (Mrs Ibstock, carer)

It is not surprising, perhaps, that Mrs Jefferson and Mr Ibstock interpreted their behaviour differently. Mrs Jefferson felt that her disability had brought her and her husband too close and that this *made* her too reliant on him. Mr Ibstock explained his wish for his wife to give up her present job as a desire to see her carrying a lighter load. However, he also said that he did not wish her to give up paid work entirely because he thought that it was important for them to have some time apart.

As well as the problems of being at home together, several respondents mentioned the related problem of not going out together socially:

> you do get at each other's throat when you're stuck in and you can't get out like you used to. I mean, we're not fantastic dancers but we used to [dance] when we went out but he can't do that now. (Mrs Mead, carer)

This issue was particularly important for those female carers who did not have an independent social life of their own and who felt uncomfortable about going out without their partner. These carers, thus, lost their own social life entirely when their husbands lost theirs (see Chapter 8).

Sexual relationship

The sexual relationship is an important part of the cement of a marriage or marriage-like relationship (Duck 1986) as well as 'an integral part of self-image and an important means of creating feelings of self-worth' (Morris 1989: 70). Almost all couples reported a change in their physical relationship and five couples were totally unable to have a full sexual relationship. Both pain and physical impairments were involved in these changes. Couples varied in the extent to which they reported being bothered or upset by the lack of a sexual relationship, and spouses and carers also varied in their views.

Mr Keighley, for example, was very distressed by his condition, not so much for himself, but for his wife's sake, after 14 years of celibacy: 'I feel very guilty in letting [wife] down regarding married life. Before this happened we had a good, happy married life . . . it [doesn't] bother me because I can't help meself. But . . . [wife]'s living like a nun and, to me, I think, well I'm letting her down' (Mr Keighley, spouse).

Mrs Keighley, by contrast, although obviously saddened by what had happened, had accommodated to the situation:

> it is no problem now, but in the beginning it was [pause] – it was more in your mind, you know [pause]. Should we, should we not, and all the rest of it, is it right, is it wrong, are you doing any harm . . . So we sort of compromised and that's it. (Mrs Keighley, carer)

Similarly, Mr and Mrs Baker expressed rather different attitudes:

> there's nothing there [sexually], put it that way. But I mean at our age we just don't, but you know. Not.
> *Interviewer: And do you think that's because of the disability or would it – ?*
> Oh yes. Definitely that. Yes. Definitely yes. But we don't, er, we don't talk like that either. You know, we never, it's never discussed. So we just get on with it. (Mrs Baker, carer)

Mr Baker appeared to be much more concerned by the loss, especially when he compared his and his wife's current situation to how they had been previously:

> when we were both working, we still thought a lot about each other and we done what other people done, thought it was one of them things that just had to be done. But now it's different you see. When you cast your mind back and say, 'Ah, it's ten years since, it's maybe ten years since, Agnes'. She says, 'Oh aye'. Now she sits down here on a night when she's watching the telly, in her nightie and her dressing gown. She wouldn't dare when we was working! Now all that's gone, she sits down there and no bother. (Mr Baker, spouse)

Other couples gave more congruent accounts of how the lack of a full sexual relationship affected them:

> that's caput like . . . I mean we make a joke about this, and we have our private little laugh about it and we keep saying, 'Never mind, but wait – one of these days!' But otherwise the relationship's just the same as it always has been. (Mrs Derby, carer)

> it must be six years since we had any contact, sort of thing, but we still, we give one another a kiss and a cuddle . . . well, I suppose time will tell . . . we've talked about it and we said, never mind, it's not everything, it'll come back. But I think it can be a bit traumatic for one or other partner when it goes over a long period like that. (Mr Derby, spouse)

The ability to talk about sexual difficulties and, in some cases, to joke about them was obviously important. There was no evidence of out and out disagreement about sexual matters between couples, but it is doubtful whether such an issue would have emerged from these interviews. However, there were hints of the difficulty that it caused for some couples, especially younger ones.

Older couples often called their age in defence of declining or ceased sexual activity, and this helped psychologically although they might still regret the loss. For younger couples this was not the case:

> In time, given time, fair enough, as you get older it's not quite so important but we're not that old yet. We're just sort of *just* middle-aged, and it's still important. Very. But we succeed now and again but, er, there are enormous problems. (Mr Jefferson, carer)

Other couples were using their age as an explanation at a much earlier stage in their lives than might have been expected.

Some wives seemed to have made a mental trade-off for the continued stability of their husbands' condition against the loss of sexual activity:

> I don't think it made a great deal of difference because, like – I was preoccupied thinking about other things really and as long as I got him back to health I wasn't really bothered . . . (Mrs Alston, carer)

> As long – if I could keep him at that stage where he is now, although it is a bad state to be at, but if I could keep him at that stage and not let him get any worse I'd be quite content, I'd be quite happy. (Mrs Ibstock, carer)

The nature of the help which carers provided for their spouses could make sexual relationships more difficult:

> sex life, that's affected you know, you have to ask your wife to do lots of things you wouldn't normally ask a wife to do . . . like when she goes out in the morning – 'Will you leave me . . . a [urine] bottle, love'. I suppose it can't be very pleasant for her. As I say, sex life is dramatically curtailed . . . (Mr Ord, spouse)

> Well some of the things I have to do are not what you describe as being very romantic, certainly not, far from it. And then to have, um, to do all those things and then try and have some kind of a normal sexual relationship can be difficult. (Mr Jefferson, carer)

All but one of the couples studied here had found their sexual relationship affected, to varying degrees, yet none had received any information or advice about how to maintain it. To a large extent spouses seemed more concerned about the loss than did carers. Spouses, who had already had so many aspects of giving – whether as breadwinners or as home-makers – taken away from them, could feel themselves further devalued by the loss of sexual giving. The Jeffersons, for example, maintained a sexual relationship, despite very difficult physical circumstances:

> I know from [wife's] point of view it's extremely important to her because it's just about the only thing that she can give back to me, she's lost so much . . .
>   I don't think that mentally she could take [the loss of their sexual relationship] because I think it would make her worse. I think she would fear even more that I was going to go off with somebody else because she would feel completely useless. (Mr Jefferson, carer)

Other couples maintained physical intimacy with a kiss and a cuddle when intercourse was impossible and this was clearly important to them. If this level of physical closeness was lost, even if it did mean less pain for the spouse, it could be devastating:

> I can't cuddle [wife] or hold her in my arms like I used to do and want to do. It's just not human for someone to lean against me with this lot [surgical corset] on me. She's afraid to hurt me, she's afraid of hurting me in any way.
>
> When I walk down the road and hold hands with her it's something out of this world. I say to her, 'We're courting', and then we realise it's just memories. (Mr Keighley, spouse)

The nature and meaning of marriage

While talking about the experience of disability in relation to their marriages, couples also said a lot about their beliefs about the nature and meaning of marriage generally. These views are important because they may help to explain why couples stay together despite considerable stresses and strains on their relationship. Without parallel information about couples who do split after one of the partners becomes ill or disabled we cannot be wholly sure about the importance of these beliefs. It may be that other couples part because of a difficult housing situation, because they cannot afford to stay together, because the disabled spouse can no longer be looked after at home and so on, rather than because they hold different views on or were differently committed to the relationship than were other couples. There is some evidence for all these triggers to marital breakdown in the existing literature on caring and disability. However, views and beliefs about marriage, as well as personality, do also influence outcomes (Dominian 1985; Mansfield and Collard 1988). There is no reason to suggest that these factors would not also be at work in marriages where disability has intervened.

Marriage as an exchange relationship

Many informal relationships between people are based on notions of exchange and reciprocity, even if these notions are rarely or never given verbal expression. Within relationships at the less close end of the spectrum, for example, between neighbours, the weighing up of giving and receiving may be quite near to the surface (see Chapter 3). By contrast, the closer the relationship, the less likely these issues are to be in the forefront of people's minds:

> in long term relationships we are . . . prepared to extend a kind of social 'hire-purchase' facility, and to do things for friends, spouses or family that we would expect to be repaid any time in the distant future, or by some other means than exact reciprocity. (Duck 1983: 108)

However, as Duck goes on to point out, when the fairness or equity of a relationship feels out of balance, 'the partners soon revert to focusing on the exchange more closely' (ibid). This focusing on the exchange has generally been ignored by commentators on informal care or, where mentioned, has been assumed not to exist in close, as opposed to more distant, relationships. Land and

Rose (1985), for example, say that in friendships between those of 'approximately equal social power, in which practical and emotional help is offered and received on a mutual basis . . . there is no invisible accountant balancing the credits and debits between the parties. And while it is not unlikely that the exchange will be more or less even, this is not predicated by the nature of the relationship' (pp. 90–91). Similarly, Jordan (1990) asserts that the 'most common approach' to 'the arrangements under which people share their lives' is of 'give and take, with frequent adaptations to crises, illnesses and emergencies, and no careful account of who owes a favour to whom, or when it should be repaid' (p. 12). Like Land and Rose, Jordan presents a rosy picture of the 'give and take' of everyday life where friends 'do not reckon up how much support or practical assistance is owed to them' (p. 14). In fact, as social psychology shows, people do keep an invisible tally of help given and received, and do attempt to redress the situation when the exchange is seen to be out of balance.

Notions of what is fair or equitable in relationships are, however, determined by social expectations and, thereby, are gender specific. (Although little of the social psychology research which Duck reports appears to take this into account.) Most important of these expectations in relation to this study is, perhaps, the breadwinner/home-maker exchange; that is, in return for the breadwinner's (usually the man's) paid labour and financial support of the household, the home-maker (usually the woman) provides unpaid domestic labour, child care and some degree of personal care for other members of the household. This is, of course, a partial, imperfect and increasingly inaccurate characterization of the relationship between men and women in marital or quasi-marital relationships. As we saw at the beginning of the chapter, however, it remains important in the study of marriage because it is a characterization which is still firmly embedded in the *ideology* of marriage (Morgan 1991). Consequently, it is strongly reflected in the accounts that men and women give of their respective roles in marital relationships, even though it may be at variance, either partial or complete, with the reality of their lives together (Oakley 1974; Mansfield and Collard 1988).

When the balance of exchange alters and equity is threatened, it is highly likely, as Duck (1983) suggests, that one or both partners will re-examine the relationship and make attempts to redress the balance. Consequently, one might expect such issues to be evident among couples who have undergone changes in the balance of their relationship. Furthermore, the greater the change, the more balancing one might expect to take place.

However, the options for redressing the balance may be severely constrained. For example, a man who was previously the main wage earner, but who becomes disabled may be denied the opportunity to provide financially, but may also be unable to, say, take on some responsibility for household tasks because of his physical impairments. Psychological constraints may also be at work; if a man's identity as the main earner is threatened his wife may be reluctant to add to that threat by becoming an earner herself and, where he is capable of doing so, asking him to do domestic tasks (Morris 1987).

When partners want to continue a relationship and when it is impossible to redress the balance by physical means, then they may attempt to alter their opinions about or evaluation of the balance itself (Duck 1983). Thus those helping a disabled spouse might ascribe more value to the relationship, as a relationship, or see their partner in a more positive light than previously. They might acknowledge the partner's *past* activities as main earner, home-maker or parent as more valuable than they would have done otherwise or feel that the imbalance in the giving/receiving equation was offset by the pain or limitations that the spouse experiences.

On the spouse's side, however, there may be less scope for psychological adjustment. Given normative emphasis on traditional role performance, the spouse may see him or herself as in debit, with few or no opportunities to change that situation. The main psychological options open to him or her may be either to devalue (or not acknowledge) the carer (and what s/he does) or to devalue him/herself. The first option could easily lead to a rapid deterioration in the relationship, while the second option might involve the carer in a lot of work boosting the spouse's opinion of him/herself to maintain the balance.

The interviews revealed views and readjustments of the sort that equity theory would predict but, as we shall see, these were often firmly based on normative beliefs both about what marriage itself was or should be about, and about men's and women's respective roles within marriage.

Revaluing the relationship and the partner

Despite the fact that all couples described some negative impact on their lives together many also said that the experience had brought them closer together or strengthened their relationship. Carers, particularly the men, were rather more likely to say this than were spouses, a finding congruent with equity theory. Carers explained this increased closeness in terms of a deeper understanding and appreciation of their spouse or as a result of increased strength through adversity:

> It helps you kind of perhaps understand each other a little better and it makes you realise . . .
> It's made me think when she's been ill, you know, more about *her* which is what we should do anyway really, well or ill, but we don't, you're too busy enjoying your life, aren't you? (Mr Quincy, carer)

> I think with the different struggles and that, if anything, it's brought us closer together. Because at certain times he's had to depend more on me but I get strength from helping him and knowing that I can be there and do little things for him and it unites you. (Mrs Alston, carer)

Carers had gone through a process of re-evaluating both their spouse and the marriage in the light of disability. Spouses, by contrast, spoke about being closer, but tended to explain this as due to the effects of having been together for a long time rather than to the disability *per se*.

Both carers and spouses compared their relationship with other, hypothetical ones which they believed could not have survived the spouse's disability in the way that theirs had. Thoughts of this sort also allowed a few carers to revalue *themselves*; not everyone, they felt, would be prepared to do what they did; therefore, they were special: 'a lot of wives wouldn't tolerate what I tolerate really, I mean I know that for a fact, and a lot just think of themselves, you know, they want to go out and that' (Mrs Gifford, carer).

The spouses who spoke of their partners in this way were women who compared what their partners did for them against what one could expect from men, in general, rather than from a husband in particular:

not many men would put up with what he's put up with. I mean he was only thirty-eight, the same age as me, I was thirty-eight when it started. How many men would put up with what he's had to put up with? (Mrs Eden, spouse)

I think you've got to be a, how can I put it, a certain calibre to be able to cope with it, because it's not all men that do . . . (Mrs Linton, spouse)

Carers also valued the ways in which their spouses dealt with their impairments and associated pain:

You have to make allowances for each other – in fact, if somebody's ill then it doesn't make them feel very happy to be ill and *you* know they try their best to keep plodding on and be as happy as they can about a raw deal. You can't turn your back on that. I couldn't. (Mrs Keighley, carer)

This process might allow both carers and spouses to feel that any apparently greater contribution the carer might make to the relationship was offset by the costs the spouse was felt to bear. As Duck has suggested, in such situations:

even if I have to put in an awful lot of effort for very small reward . . . I may nevertheless feel that the relationship is equitable because the friend has to suffer so much more to receive the perhaps slightly greater rewards. In this case our rewards might not be equal but neither are the costs and efforts, and we shall both still feel that the relationship is an equitable one that we wish to preserve. (Duck 1986: 109)

However, it was important that valuing the spouse should not tip over into pity, because that would change the nature of the relationship in a very fundamental way: 'I haven't started to feel pity for him yet. I mean the love and that is still there but I think if I ever did start to feel pity I think I would just end it like, I wouldn't carry on' (Mrs Ibstock, carer).

Reciprocity and duty

Another psychological approach to balancing a relationship in which the partners' relative inputs and outputs are perceived to be out of kilter is to refer to reciprocity. Some carers said that they looked after their spouses either because they believed that their spouses would have looked after them, had their positions been reversed, or because they had actually done so at some time in the past. Others pointed to the on-going emotional support that their spouses could provide, even if they could not contribute practically:

For all that [I am protective of him] I can sit down and lean on him for a lot of other things, he's so down to earth and if I've anything wrong and I'm worrying about it, about meself, and I tell him, [he says] 'That's nowt', you know, he can smooth it over and make me feel a lot better. (Mrs Derby, carer)

Then there were those carers who saw what they did as being, in some sense, a repayment for the spouse's having been 'a good husband' or 'a good wife':

I had him spoilt because I thought, oh, he's got what he's got. I mean he's been good to the kids and to me and that and I thought, oh it's a shame. (Mrs Ibstock, carer)

You don't get married and raise five kiddies to wipe your hands of somebody that's poorly. Well I don't anyway, it's not my way . . . I've put some hard work into this marriage, but the wife has also because apart from her suffering like she has suffered she's still done her job, she's still done her duty, she's still been a good wife, but it must have been hard for her with her being the one that suffers. (Mr Linton, carer)

Here we can see that notions of reciprocation sometimes came very close to notions of doing right or of duty. The spouse had played his or her part according to the rules; therefore, the carer felt that he or she had a responsibility or duty to do the same.

Just over half of the carers, and similar proportions of men and women, spoke of their duty or responsibility to care. This suggests that, at least within the bounds of marriage, differences between female and male carers are not as great as previous work on informal care might have suggested (Ungerson 1987).

Statements about duty and responsibility were rarely made within an overtly cultural framework. Mr Uckfield said that it was his religious and moral duty to care for his wife and would clearly have been shocked had any other arrangement been suggested to him. Others were less clear about from where this incentive came – one just did it and got on with it:

He's my responsibility and that's it. And, um, I just couldn't leave him to anyone else anyway. (Mrs Baker, carer)

I don't know what it is, whether it's being pig-headed or what, I don't know really. I feel it's me duty while [wife]'s not well and I feel it's me duty to do it, you see, and that's it. (Mr Eden, carer)

I look at it this way, maybe I'm old fashioned but, I don't know, but she's my wife and I'll look after her, I don't care what happens . . . whilst she's with me I'll do whatever I can for her. (Mr Linton, carer)

Carers were not usually able to say clearly from where this moral imperative to help came, but it seemed to be deeply embedded within their system of beliefs about marriage and the responsibilities that being married entailed. Several people referred to 'others' who, they believed, would not be as committed as they were and whose marriages, therefore, would be less likely to survive.

Spouse's self-esteem

Spouses' strategies for balancing up perceived inequities within the marriage were often more limited than those available to carers. The interviews revealed a substantial subgroup – mostly, but not exclusively, amongst the most disabled spouses – who expressed feelings of sadness or even guilt at what they saw as the limitations their disability imposed on the carer's life. Some spouses clung to this devaluation of themselves even when their carer tried to persuade them otherwise:

I say things to her like, 'You know, Agnes, you're not leading a normal life, you should be leading a different life'. She says, 'I'm happy, I'm happy. If you're happy, I'm happy' . . . (Mr Baker, spouse)

Carers were often involved in trying to boost the spouse's opinion of him or herself. Furthermore, they were often hurt themselves by their spouse's feelings of low self-esteem, particularly when this led to the spouse suggesting that the carer would be better off without him or her:

> it hurts, you know, he'll say, 'I'm just a nuisance', this kind of thing, so you have to sort of jolly him out of it, if you like. (Mrs Keighley, carer)

Female spouses were more likely to express sadness or guilt about the burden they felt they imposed on their partners than were male spouses. Moreover, while it was the most seriously disabled husbands who expressed these feelings, among the female spouses there was no apparent association between the degree of disability and such feelings. As argued earlier, this must be explained in some degree by the very visible difference between what men normally do and what they do when they become carers. By contrast, the difference between what women normally do and what they do as carers is less obvious. Consequently, male spouses notice the imbalance in the normal give and take of the relationship only when it is very pronounced while female spouses notice it much earlier. Furthermore, when women are so well trained to be givers rather than receivers, it is not surprising that they find shifts in the balance of giving and taking more difficult to cope with (Gilligan 1982).

This is another area, then, in which the perception of equity and inequity in marital relationships is influenced substantially by social expectation and, there-fore, also by gender. However, the differences in how female and male spouses felt about this imbalance were not paralleled by differences between male and female carers. As we have seen carers used other psychological techniques for redressing perceived imbalances.

Some spouses identified ways in which they contributed to the relationship and thus could feel that the relationship was more balanced. Mr Alston and Mr Keighley, for example, planned their finances to ensure that their wives would be 'all right' financially should they die (see Chapter 5). Other male spouses, par-ticularly those who were most disabled, tried to help out around the home, while female spouses fought to maintain their role as home-maker for as long as they could. For a few seriously disabled spouses, however, there was little they felt they could do, either practically or financially, to 'compensate' their partners; all they could look to was luck:

> I would like to help her like I used to and I can't do it and when I get into one of my moods I say, 'Why the hell should she have to do everything' and I'm not doing nowt to help her and that's when it gets me down. But other times I bear meself up and I say, well, you're lucky that she's there to do for you or you'd be in an old people's home or something.
>
> My view is, she's my number one. Come the treble chance I might take her to Switzerland. (Mr Baker, spouse)

Thoughts on separation and divorce

By definition, the group of people interviewed in this study were 'very married'. Their relationships had continued after the onset of the spouse's disability for periods of at least four years and, for many, far longer. By a purely operational definition, then, these marriages were strong. However, strength – especially in relation to emotional relationships – is not a singular concept. People may remain together, despite substantial strains, because they love one another, because they feel that it is their duty to remain together, or because circumstances force them to stay together when they might rather part.

Furthermore, the strength of a relationship has a temporal quality, stronger at some times than at others. For example, research has shown that marriages are particularly vulnerable after the birth of the first child (Dominian 1985). However, that these couples were still married does not mean that they had never considered separating or that they might not do so in the future. Indeed, one or both partners in a third of the couples said that they had already contemplated ending the marriage.

In a few instances thoughts of leaving arose from problems in the relationship which had existed prior to the spouse's disability. However, the disability had made an already difficult situation even worse:

> What suits you at twenty doesn't suit you when you get to fifty, does it? You don't grow together, I think you grow away . . .
> I was so used to having him away at sea, I was so used to standing on my own two feet that I think I most likely would have walked out and have a life of my own, once the children had gone. (Mrs Eden, spouse)

Similarly Mr and Mrs Fowey had always had a stormy relationship, and Mrs Fowey had actually left home in the early years of their marriage. The onset of Mr Fowey's heart disease and colitis had, however, made things a lot worse, particularly when he left paid work and spent most of his day at home.

In reality both these women were constrained by all that they would lose if they left home and the difficulties of replacing it:

> I thought, well, I worked for the biggest part of my home – I paid the bills, the gas, electric, the phone bill and anything the kids wanted I used to buy them. I think, well, for what I've got I've had to work bloody hard for, and why should I leave it? (Mrs Fowey, carer)

In addition, for Mrs Fowey, there was the worry about 'what might happen' if she were to leave her husband: 'I thought if I leave him and he dies, you know, I'll feel guilty or if he took any worse I'd feel guilty and my duty was beside him when he was bad . . .'.

Thus, while both these women experienced practical constraints on their ability to leave home and become independent, Mrs Fowey had the additional constraint of a feeling of duty towards her husband which was, apparently, triggered by his being ill. Had he not been ill, she implied, she would have left, especially as the children were now grown.

In other cases thoughts of leaving home or ending the marriage had occurred only since the onset of the spouse's disability and in direct response to it. In most of these couples the spouse was substantially disabled. In all instances where spouses talked about this issue they spoke in terms of having offered to leave, to relieve their carers of the burden they felt they imposed:

> I would have rather done that [gone into residential care] and still been friends than to drag her down and drag her down to such a point where we argued and got on each other's nerves and fought and *had* to break up, you know, *forced* to break up and

broke up not being friends. I would have rather had it that way, the first way, than the second way, but no, she wouldn't have that. (Mr Ibstock, spouse)

over the years, I said, I wouldn't blame her, she could go out on me any time, I wouldn't blame her. I said, I'm no good in any way to her, only a burden. (Mr Keighley, spouse)

It is not at all clear that spouses expected these offers to be taken up. While they could act as a signal to the carers that they were free to go if they wanted to, the offers can also be seen as ways in which the spouse could confirm that s/he was still valuable to the carer: 'I thought it would be better [to go and live in a home] but of course [wife] didn't see it that way. She says, no, we got married for better or worse, that's it' (Mr Ibstock, spouse).

Spouses, then, offered to leave or to let the carer off her/his obligations. Carers thought about leaving when the responsibilities just became too much: 'I've walked out and I've walked around and perhaps gone and seen a friend of mine or something like that, sat and talked . . . I think your system can only take so much and then it reacts, whether you like it or not' (Mr Jefferson, carer).

However, there were powerful constraints against separating, not least of which were, again, practical. For example, as Mr Ord (a spouse) pointed out in his interview, even if he and his wife had wanted to separate they could not have afforded to do so. Carers themselves thought more in terms of who would look after their spouse if they went and also in terms of their duty towards or affection for their spouse:

Interviewer: Have you ever thought about putting your coat on and going?
[Pause] Then, yes [when husband was first disabled], but not now. It would have been very easy then.
*Interviewer: Then somebody else would have **had** to do something?*
Yes, they would.
Interviewer: What stopped you doing that?
He's my husband, and I love him, so, that's it. (Mrs Ord, carer)

As Mrs Ord's quotations suggests, some couples had experienced times in the past when their relationship had been under greater strain than it was at the time of the interview. This was true not only for those who had ever contemplated separation, but for several others too. These others recognized that, in different circumstances – with different people involved or if the strain had continued – then their marriage could have been in jeopardy: 'if our marriage had been, you know, tilting a little bit when he had this accident, I don't think we would have survived. I don't think we would because it's been a trying time . . .' (Mrs Hazleton, carer).

Marriages were often under the greatest strain at the time when the disability started or became substantially worse. Most couples were left more or less entirely unsupported at this time (see Chapter 4), and had to make many psychological and practical adjustments to their lives with little help or advice. More by their own efforts than by help from outside, they had survived an extremely difficult period of their lives with their marriages intact.

Conclusions

In this chapter we have catalogued some of the ways in which couples felt that their marriage had been affected. They reported increased bad temper (on both sides of the relationship), the strains of being together too much, and the very substantial effects that impairment had had on their physical relationship.

Given that so much of their experience was negative, what kept these couples together? Furthermore, can we learn anything from their experiences about what might cause other marriages to break up?

There seemed to be five main factors which affected the nature of these couples' marriages and, thus, the likelihood of their staying together. Some of these factors were interdependent and it is not at all clear which, if any, was more important than any other.

First, and most obviously perhaps, was the quality of the marriage before the onset of disability. Many respondents reported that they had always had a close relationship and those that had not were the ones whose marriages seemed the least happy at the time of being interviewed. The affection that some couples felt for one another despite, and in some cases perhaps because of, all they had gone through was almost palpable during parts of the interviews. When everything else seemed to be against them such couples could rely on their love for one another to support them.

When affection failed, or had never been strong, notions of duty towards the disabled spouse, or the rightness of continuing with the marriage, come what may, kept others together. Indeed, sometimes this sense of duty was triggered or strengthened by the spouse's disability.

Thirdly, there was the severity of the spouse's disability. Even in relationships where there had been a great deal of affection, when the carer was providing a substantial amount of physical care strain in the marriage was likely.

Severity was also related to the fourth factor – time. Carrying a heavy responsibility for care-giving over a long period of time could be very destructive to relationships, especially if accompanied by changed behaviour on the spouse's part. However, some couples found that things improved with time; their marriages had been most at risk at the time when the spouse had first become disabled or when his or her condition had suddenly deteriorated. As time had gone by, even if the spouse's condition had not improved, couples had adjusted and the relationship had regained some sense of balance. However, it seems likely that the ability or willingness to hang on to the marriage during these difficult periods would itself be influenced by the original quality of the relationship or the sense of duty which the carer felt.

Finally, practical considerations also affected whether couples stayed married. For example, in the absence of adequate supportive services for disabled people, the disabled partner would, in most cases, find it difficult to replace the carer's help with daily living and the carer, particularly if a woman, would find it difficult to replace the disabled partner's income, albeit that the income might be from benefits. Finding alternative accommodation would certainly be no easier than for any separating couple and, for the disabled partner, would almost inevitably be more difficult. Thus, even if no other factor served to keep couples together, practical constraints might. Conversely, it is easy to imagine that certain types of practical considerations could contribute to driving some couples apart; difficult housing conditions, living in an isolated area and having difficulty making ends meet are a few possible examples.

All these five factors were evident, to some degree, in the lives of the couples interviewed. However, it was not uncommon for several to be at work at the same time. Thus, couples who felt a great deal of affection for one another might also have strong views about the rightness of remaining married. At the same time the spouse's level of disability and the length of time for which s/he had needed help might combine to weigh against the original strength of the relationship.

The psychological balancing of equity within the marriage is an integral part to the process of staying married. Marriages may become untenable when one or both partners *feel* that the balance is not right, not when some objective assessment suggests that it is not. As we have seen, carers possibly had more opportunities to use psychological balancing mechanisms if they chose to; so they might perceive the situation to be more equitable than did their partners. However, we have also seen that notions of equity are influenced by social expectations; consequently, men and women could be expected to have different perceptions of what is and is not equitable in their marriages.

It is not possible to legislate for happiness in marriage. It *is* possible, however, to make sure that couples who encounter impairment in their married lives are adequately supported (especially at onset or at predictably difficult times), that spouse carers do not carry heavy physical and emotional responsibilities without help or respite, that couples do not lose their sexual relationship through ignorance, embarrassment or not knowing whom to approach for help, and that couples are not bound within an empty shell of a marriage for want of practical alternatives to their current situation.

Children, disability and caring

Introduction

Evidence about whether or not, and to what degree, children experience any long-term effects when a parent becomes disabled whilst the child is growing up is hard to find. Most research in this area is characterized by anecdotal accounts and uncontrolled case-studies. The small amount of adequately designed research on the topic has suggested that adjustment in adulthood is not adversely affected by a childhood spent with a disabled parent. However, this work has tended to concentrate on one particular type of traumatically caused impairment (often spinal cord injury) rather than progressive conditions, and to investigate only families where it is the father who is disabled (see Buck and Hohmann 1983, for a review of this area).

Parents with spinal cord injuries are often separated from their children for many months, sometimes for longer than a year, during treatment and rehabilitation at spinal injury units. This period of separation can cause difficulties, particularly when children are very young. However, once relationships are re-established, and as long as the disabled parent, and his or her partner where there is one, are adequately supported, evidence suggests that children adapt rapidly to the changed circumstances (Morris 1989; Hoad *et al.* 1990; Creek *et al.* not dated).

By contrast, parents with conditions which require frequent or repeated absences from home for treatment, or which lead to rapid deterioration of the parent's physical abilities, or which are unpredictable in their progress, or which involve changes in the parent's personality, may lead to very different outcomes. The opportunities for re-establishing stable relationships in such circumstances may be much reduced (Coughlan and Humphrey 1982; Locker 1983). However, it is also possible that more gradual change, sometimes associated with progressive conditions, such as multiple sclerosis or Parkinson's disease, may make readjustment for children easier.

Another important distinction in this area is that between parenting – that is the concern that parents have for their child's welfare in all its various manifestations – and parental activity – the things that parents *do* as parents. The existing literature contains nothing to suggest that physical disability affects parents' desire or ability to parent. As Morris (1989) points out, when describing the experience of spinally injured women, 'Many of us find that, even while lying flat on our backs in hospital, we are the ones who have to organise to keep the family together and cared for' (p. 127).

By contrast, in the absence of adequate support services, disability may well affect disabled parents' parental *activity*. Disabled women describe the physical barriers to child care activities that they experience (Sainsbury 1970; Morris 1989), while disabled men (and disabled women who are single parents) report worrying about their loss of role as main earner, and the impact that this has on their children's social and recreational activities (Sainsbury 1970; Morris 1989; Hoad *et al*. 1990). Again Morris (1989) makes this distinction clear:

> It is the inaccessible parts of the home which handicap a paraplegic mother rather than the wheelchair itself. For a tetraplegic woman, having the use of someone else's hands to do what she cannot do herself enables her to look after her children. (p. 128)

The lack of adequate support for disabled parents, particularly mothers, can lead to their children being taken into care (Locker 1983) or non-disabled fathers being given custody of children after divorce (Morris 1989). Prejudice from both professionals and the world at large can also contribute to disabled women being denied the right to parent their children (Sainsbury 1970; Morris 1989).

As the above suggests, another important issue for children may be the sex of the disabled parent and, hence, that of the spouse. We saw in Chapter 5 that when a father is disabled the household's economic circumstances, although significantly reduced, may nonetheless be better than when it is a mother who is disabled. Furthermore, normative expectations about responsibility for child care may leave the children of disabled fathers potentially relatively less affected than those of disabled mothers (Sainsbury 1970). Whilst the wives of disabled men may increase their paid work to compensate for their household's reduced earnings, they are likely to continue their child caring activities. In this they are little different from many married women who carry dual responsibilities for child care and for earning. They may be less able to call on their husbands for substitute domestic or child care labour, but, again, in this they may be little different from women with non-disabled husbands. When it is the mother who is disabled, existing child care arrangements may be substantially disrupted and, where the mother is ill as well as disabled, never restored. Examples in the existing literature of children entering local authority care because of a parent's disability are all of situations where it was the mother who was disabled (Sainsbury 1970; Locker 1983; Morris 1989). Often this is associated with inadequate support in the form of substitute child care at home, or is found in the absence of flexible arrangements for fathers which would allow them to care for their children *and* maintain paid work (Blaxter 1976).

Furthermore, when mothers rather than fathers are disabled, children may be more often pulled into providing substitute domestic care, in particular if the father continues his paid work (Grimshaw 1991). Given the early age at which girls are socialized into domestic and 'caring' roles (Sharpe 1976), it also seems probable that they might find themselves involved more than boys. The gender of the child *and* that of the disabled parent, therefore, may also be important in determining whether or not parental disability has any effect on the child's life.

A final important distinction in this area is between the effects on children of having a disabled parent, and the effects on disabled parents and their partners of having children. As already suggested, once the situation stabilizes after the onset of a parent's disability, and assuming adequate support is available, young children, in particular, seem to adjust rapidly. Parents themselves, however, may continue to experience child-related effects for many years. The existing literature refers to the regret, and sometimes guilt, that both mothers and fathers can feel about their inability to do the things with their children which they feel that other mothers and fathers could. Furthermore, some couples may decide to limit family size for both practical and financial reasons when one parent has become disabled (Sainsbury 1970).

In summary, there are complex sets of inter-relating factors which *may* influence whether or not a child is affected, both in the short and the long term, by a parent being disabled. There is no conclusive evidence one way or the other, and much of the existing information relies on parents' rather than children's own reports.

Perceived effects on the children's lives

All but one of the couples interviewed had children, but only 14 of them had any of their children still at home with them at the time of the interview. An even smaller number had children who were still dependent on them. However, some other couples' children had still been at home and/or dependent when the spouse's disability or illness had started. It was on these couples, that is those whose children had been or were still dependent at the time the spouse had become disabled, that this chapter concentrates.

This section of the research was least satisfactory from a methodological view point. In all other respects people were talking about their own experiences; in this section they were talking about somebody else's. They were, of course, able to talk about what they noticed about their own relationships with the children, and the perceived effects of disability and caring on them. However, there is no way in which they could give a full account of how their children experienced this themselves.

Loss of activities

The effect on children's lives most frequently mentioned by couples was the loss of certain activities which the spouse (and sometimes the carer) would otherwise have shared with their children. This effect, however, appeared to be limited exclusively to male spouses or carers and was usually seen as most affecting sons. Playing football or cricket, taking children to football matches, teaching them how to swim, and teaching them gardening or household maintenance skills, were most often mentioned:

> [son] plays rugby. When he first started playing rugby I used to go *every* weekend with him to watch him, but I can't now . . . (Mr Rutland, spouse)

> The amount I have to do for [wife] takes up a lot of the time that I would like to have had with the boys . . . I mean, I like to go swimming, I would like to have gone with me sons . . . (Mr Jefferson, carer)

However, spouses were able to make up for their loss of physical activity with their children by spending time with them in other ways:

> He does spend more time [with daughter]. Like in a morning, he's laid out and he's got heat wrap on and he always reads – they always have about ten minutes, quarter of an hour before she goes to school. She reads to him. Things like that he can do I don't get much time for . . . (Mrs Gifford, carer)

> I think perhaps his dad has got a lot more time for him, time wise, than what, perhaps, a lot of dads have for children. Like, when he was quite little my husband was upset that he couldn't take him playing football. But I mean, you see lots of fathers that are fit, *they* don't take their sons playing football neither. So I just keep telling him this, you're giving him time. I think that has paid off. (Mrs Ord, carer)

The effects of disability could also spread over into the next generation and affect the things that older couples were able to do with their grandchildren. This perhaps was a more significant loss for the grandparents than it was for their grandchildren:

> we used to take them in the car – take them over to the Lake District or something. We used to stop over there for the weekend with them . . . walk them up the mountains and that . . . and now if we do take them anywhere [it's less energetic] . . .
>
>   We go on a green like, to a picnic . . . and I just read my paper or have five minutes shut eye [while grandchildren explore] . . . but when they come to play football and things like that and there are people playing with their granddad's football and that, and they just play football [without me]. (Mr Ibstock, spouse)

Restrictions on mobility and the time taken up looking after a spouse meant that some people did not get to see their grandchildren at all, unless they came to visit. Mrs Baker, for example, had not seen her youngest daughter's first child until several weeks after the birth. Furthermore, because she could not leave Mr Baker for any length of time, she had been unable to help her daughter out during the time after the birth in the way she might otherwise have done.

Taking a back seat

While spouses spoke more about restrictions in the physical activities they could share with their children, carers were more likely to talk about the children having to take a back seat to the spouse's needs. When this happened carers themselves felt that they were less involved with their children's lives: 'sometimes [she]'ll take a back seat. If she wants something but [husband] wants the attention if he's really bad, she'll just have to wait while I'm seeing to him' (Mrs Gifford, carer).

As we saw above, in some families the spouse could compensate by taking more time with the child. In others, the carer would make an extra effort with the child during any periods when the spouse's needs were less:

> She does have less time to spend with [daughter] but she does make up for it. She tries to make up for it . . . she likes to get her involved in things that she's interested in,

when she can . . . the best is when she takes her to town shopping with her . . . and she finds shopping with [wife] very interesting. Because she'll come back and she'll say, we enjoyed that trip to town and they seem to be really chummy when they go to town shopping . . . (Mr Gifford, spouse)

Some couples, when they were able to, made up in material goods for other things that they felt their children missed:

[Her father] does other things for her . . . after his dad died his mum gave [daughter] her old stereo thing – she's lucky really, she's got all that upstairs . . . [husband] just put her a shelf up and set it her all up. She's got a little telly but it were only what his dad had . . . So people might think, 'God, she's got this, that, other' but it's only what she's come in line for . . . I couldn't afford to go out and buy her a £400 stereo, no way. So this year she's after a colour telly, she is, for Christmas. So we're hoping to be able to get her one. (Mrs Gifford, carer, daughter is 9)

While these parents seemed to be trying to compensate their child in material ways other couples, who had more than one child, felt that their children had suffered because of the general lack of money. There was less money around for things that their contemporaries might have, fewer holidays and so on. Most children, especially those old enough to understand the reasons for it, were said to be reasonable about such financial restrictions but, for some at least, there was residual resentment:

when Dad gave up work I think they realised that we just had to draw our wings in somewhere. I mean we never spread them that much but when the main one has to give up working you've got to do something about it. (Mrs Clifton, carer)

of course [they've been affected] financially as well. Oh, you know, so and so, his mum and dad . . . helped him get a car, and they're doing this, well we can't, we can't do it. I'm not saying it's a bad thing for kids to have to try and get these things on their own, I think it's a good thing . . . but it would be nice to [help them out financially] if you could do it. We can't really because whatever finances we have had, have to help support our situation. (Mr Jefferson, carer)

Emotional effects

Although parents mostly talked about practical and financial effects on their children some were also able to point to emotional effects, such as worry and anxiety around the spouse's disability and its perceived effects:

[daughter] used to worry about him . . . Once she knew that was the finish, he couldn't go back to work any more. She once said to me, 'What are we going to do, Mummy?' (Mrs Hazleton, carer)

it has had some effect on them. It does make them sad, you know, when one of us is ill and we've noticed that. They do get very concerned in their own little way and I think people tend to forget that, that children aren't children, they're only small adults and they think and act just like we do. And it does have an effect on them because you can tell they are different when you're both well, when you're bouncing, they're bouncing . . . (Mr Quincy, carer)

This last quotation is particularly important because although Mrs Quincy was disabled both partners had been severely ill at different times in the recent past. It was in this family where there had been the most obvious effects on the children, particularly the elder one. Mrs Quincy had been very depressed after the birth of the younger child and the elder, her daughter, had taken on a great deal of responsibility around the house, and for the baby, although she was only six years old at the time. Later on, after her husband and her son had both been ill, Mrs Quincy had become depressed again and the children had had to spend a month with their grandparents. Both had then started bed-wetting. The daughter had started to have migraine attacks and was often reluctant to go to school:

> she's never liked school. And I was told by the health visitor . . . she says, you're too close for good. I says, what do you mean? She says, look at her, hanging on to you, clinging on. I mean, fair enough, she was nine, 'cos this is only a couple of years ago the health visitor came out to say this . . . [daughter] had the spell of wetting her bed and [the health visitor] turned round and said, you're pampering her . . . Obviously she didn't know my circumstances, and [daughter] was there – and [she] just turned round to her and said, 'You don't know anything about my mum or me'. You know she thinks . . . her thinking's very grown up. Whether it has to be, you know. But I find she likes to be at home with me . . . I do tend to make her go to school but if she can she'll spend the time with me. (Mrs Quincy, spouse)

Young children, particularly, needed some sense of constancy and when both parents were ill or incapacitated this could disappear. Mr Gifford explained how important this reassurance was for his young daughter:

> I wouldn't say she worries too much. She might seem concerned sometimes when I'm in a lot of pain. She'll seem concerned but I wouldn't say she worries – not to that extent – because she knows that we cope with it. She knows that *we* are able to cope with it so she's confident that we can get over that problem . . . If she thought that we couldn't cope with it she probably would [worry]. But she knows that we can.

The Quincy's children, by contrast, had gone through a very traumatic period when neither parent was 'coping with it', with consequent emotional effects. The Quincy's had received no practical or, indeed, emotional support from formal services during these very difficult periods in their life. Consequently, the daughter had carried a substantial burden of practical and emotional responsibility at a very young age:

> it's something she has had to do . . . it's been a responsibility for her . . . as she is my responsibility, I sometimes become her responsibility. You know and she knows this and she's fully aware of the circumstances and everything . . . (Mrs Quincy, spouse)

Mental health problems, such as Mrs Quincy's, or changes in personality associated with a disability, were clearly more difficult for children to cope with emotionally than were physical disabilities. Mr and Mrs Jefferson's elder son, for example, had found Mrs Jefferson's increasingly difficult personality, brought on by progressive brain damage, very hard to come to terms with and had eventually left home:

he would see me doing everything I possibly could and still be in trouble, if you like, and he would just say, 'Mum, for God's sake leave me Dad alone, he's done every-thing he can' . . . and then she'd probably turn on him you see . . .

He's very quiet, I've known times . . . he's a big lad, he's six foot one . . . and he's thick set. And I've known times, I've come past that room and he's been crying his eyes out and sometimes I've just left him, sometimes I've sat on the end of his bed and talked to him about it and try to explain as best I can why his mum acts the way she does . . . (Mr Jefferson, carer)

Both carers and spouses could be aware of the emotional effects that their children might experience and do their best to protect them. Mrs Quincy, for example, hid a lot from her younger child because she thought he dealt with it less well than did his older sister: 'I've never hid anything from [daughter]. I have to do from [son] because he's different . . . not because he's so young, not because he's a boy or anything like that, it's the fact that he can't cope in the same way somehow.'

Mr Gifford was similarly reluctant to involve his young daughter too much because he felt that she was too young:

She may be able to help me more as she gets older with things, she's probably more aware of things but you see, you can't put, I don't like to put too old a head on her, not at nine year old – they've got to go through their childhood, and they should go through it properly, so I don't like to overload her mind with things that she shouldn't be bothered with at the moment.

As we shall see again later in the chapter the child's age, particularly at the time the parent had first become disabled or sick, seemed to parents to be important in influencing how children reacted.

Becoming more understanding and helpful

Not all, nor even the majority, of the effects of having a parent who becomes disabled while the child is still young are negative ones then. We have already seen that disabled parents felt that they were able to spend more time with their children. Couples spontaneously reported other positive effects, particularly in relation to children's increased understanding and general helpfulness.

Moreover, even though some children might become more involved in helping out at home or might miss activities that other children shared with their parents, most managed to stay just like other children: 'I would say he's just like an average 12 year old boy, well what I would expect an average 12 year old boy to be like . . .'. (Mr Ord, spouse)

Age of the children and nature of the parents' impairments

Couples were quite clear that the age of their children at the time when the parent's impairments had started or significantly worsened was of great import-ance in determining the way they reacted to it. For example, most of those whose children were well into their teens at the time felt that there had been little observable effect:

Interviewer: All the children were pretty much grown up before you were much affected by your illness?
Oh yeah. It hasn't affected their lives. It only affected their lives that I can't go and see them. (Mr Baker, spouse) . . .

Our [elder son] was 15, 16 at the time. Well, I think at 15 and 16 they're more interested in their own lives really, aren't they? As long as he didn't have to help me *too* much and he could get out with his mates at that age . . . (Mrs Rutland, carer)

Parents of children who had been very young felt that they, too, were little affected because they had grown up with it:

he was only three weeks old [when father became disabled] so like he's always grown up with his dad not so well. And his dad taking tablets, and in and out of hospital and up and down with the ambulance coming. So he's always known that, and I think that's probably been quite good really, whereas if it was dad taken ill now, at this age, it might have a different effect on him. (Mrs Ord, carer)

Furthermore, it was not just the age of the children, but also the *nature* of the onset of impairment that determined if and how the children were affected. Coming to terms with a parent's gradual loss of physical faculties over the years seemed to be a very different proposition from the sudden adjustment required when loss was caused by an accident or a rapidly deteriorating condition. Similarly, a sudden drop in income or change in the parent's status as breadwinner or home-maker were more likely to be difficult to cope with.

Disability and family size

Couples whose children were still young when the spouse had become disabled were asked whether they had subsequently decided to limit the size of their family. Four of the eight couples whose children had been under the age of ten at the start of the spouse's disability had made a conscious decision not to have any more children. Money and the additional responsibilities that another child would mean for the carer were the two main reasons given by these couples.

Mr and Mrs Alston already had a large family (which included children from Mr Alston's first marriage) and it had been some time before they had made the decision to have no more children. Their religious beliefs had made it a particularly difficult decision for them:

I had this agonizing decision to make. I thought, well, I'm getting to the stage [where] I'm not getting any help bringing the family up, because my husband wasn't capable, no matter how willing he was . . . I could see the future coming where he wouldn't be able to support the family, not to go out to work. And I thought, well, I can't really settle for taking the chance of whether I would have any more family or not . . . (Mrs Alston, carer)

Mr and Mrs Gifford had lost their first baby and had their daughter fairly soon afterwards. They had originally wanted to have two children, but with Mr Gifford's increasing impairments they decided against it:

it'd have been silly, just to add more work on to me . . .

As it happens, with [husband] getting worse over years, it's been a good thing really. It would have been more work on me still and I've enough on me plate. (Mrs Gifford, carer)

Both Mr and Mrs Ord emphasized the financial impact of having another child as their reason for not increasing their family size, but for Mrs Ord the additional responsibility it would have placed on her was also important:

We just thought well we couldn't really afford to have another child. It's not very nice to keep saying to children, no, all the time . . . so we just settled for one . . .

I think that probably it is as well that [son] came early, even before my husband got bad, or else I don't think we would have had any children.

Interviewer: You don't think you would?

I don't think so, no. I think it would be very awkward to try and cope with a baby and [husband] so I think perhaps it was as well that [son] was born when he was born. (Mrs Ord, carer)

With the fourth couple it was difficult to judge whether they might have contemplated having more children, but Mr Jefferson had taken an apparently unilateral decision to have a vasectomy as soon as his wife's multiple sclerosis was diagnosed. He did not actually talk about this during his interview; it was Mrs Jefferson who brought the subject up. It seems that they might have had another child if Mrs Jefferson had not become ill (the younger was only four and the elder nine at the time), but Mr Jefferson was not, in any case, prepared to risk the possibility of Mrs Jefferson's becoming pregnant.

It is difficult to know what the long-term effect of restricting family size because of a parent's disability might be. On the one hand, one can see that existing children might be enabled to live a life more like that of their peers, especially in regard to material goods, if family size is not increased. She or he is also likely to receive more attention from both spouse and carer. On the other hand, the fewer children there are in the family the greater the responsibility those children might have to carry in the future, particularly if the carer becomes ill or frail her/himself. Responsibility for, particularly, elderly parents does not currently fall equally on all children, but if there *is* only one child then there is little or no choice for that child. Furthermore, the more adult children there are, the more likely material help is to be forthcoming (see Chapter 3). As long as the carer is alive and well, or the marriage survives then the child, on the evidence of these interviews at least, seems to be protected from becoming too involved in caring. Anecdotal evidence suggests that when the carer-parent goes, in the absence of supportive services, only children are particularly vulnerable to becoming carers themselves (Leventon and Jeffries 1988).

Conclusions

Having a disabled parent was acknowledged by couples to have affected younger children to some degree. They lost the opportunity to share activities with their parents which other children enjoy, they occasionally had to take a back seat to the disabled parent's needs, and they had experienced a level of anxiety and worry in their everyday lives that other children do not. However, most of the couples worked hard to protect their children and positive effects were evident too. Difficulties arose, however, when this protection broke down, perhaps because the carer-parent became ill. Furthermore, if the onset of disability was sudden or deterioration was rapid, and the child was at a certain age, then the impact on the child could be more significant than in other situations. There is also a suggestion that mental health problems or personality changes were more likely to have an effect.

There was no evidence, apart from the one case where both parents had been ill, of children becoming over-involved in providing care themselves. They perhaps helped out a little more around the house and were more sympathetic to the spouse's needs than they would otherwise have been. For the most part, however, their parents strove to make their lives as normal as possible and in some circumstances to compensate them, materially or with attention, for what few losses that they were felt to experience. However, some couples had to make difficult decisions about restricting their family size so that they could maintain as much normality as possible. This was a real and significant loss for the couples and possibly, in the long term, for the children themselves.

It says much about the financial situation of such couples and about the lack of practical support they received that disability had such an effect on the choices they had to make about their lives.

It hurts more inside:
being a spouse carer

Introduction

The bulk of this book has been concerned with the effect of disability on married *couples*. Throughout we have examined both the spouse's and the carer's views and experiences. In this chapter we shall concentrate rather more on the carer, looking at the responsibilities and restrictions that caring for a spouse in the absence of supportive services brings. Just as spouse carers carry out caring tasks similar to those undertaken by other sorts of carers, so the restrictions and responsibilities they experience are similar to those documented in studies of other groups of carers. However, there may be aspects of caring for a spouse which are not evident in other caring relationships or which are different in nature and extent. Some of these arise from the nature of the marital relationship itself (see Chapter 6), while others are a function of the position which married couples occupy in relation to, say, the provision of help and support from other informal and formal sources (see Chapters 3 and 4). Consequently, in some degree at least, the experience of caring for a spouse may be different from that of caring for any other relative.

This chapter examines both those aspects of caring which spouse carers share with other carers and those which appear to be unique to their situation. We start by examining the extent to which carers could leave the home and the impact that this had on their lives.

Time off from caring

One of the most persistent findings to emerge from the literature on informal caring, regardless of the person being cared for, is the unremitting nature of the help which has to be provided when disabled people are unsupported in any other way (e.g. Glendinning 1983; Levin *et al.* 1983; Hicks 1988). Being an informal carer to the most disabled people constitutes a job which last for 24 hours a day, 365 days of the year. Even when caring for less disabled people, the unpredictability of their condition or the need to keep an eye on them can still affect the carer's ability to lead a life of his or her own. Yet time away from the disabled person can be one of the most significant factors in reducing stress levels among carers (Bradshaw and Lawton 1976; Levin *et al.* 1983).

For a variety of reasons one might have expected the group of carers described in this study to be more able to take time off from caring than other groups already described in the literature. First, the range of impairments was wider in this study than perhaps has been the case in other small-scale research. Secondly, all the people being helped were adults and, thus, if not severely physically disabled, might have been able to be left alone. This is in contrast with caring for young children who, regardless of whether or not they are disabled, cannot be left alone for any length of time. Thirdly, with one exception, none of the spouses had such a substantial level of mental impairment that it was dangerous for them to be left even briefly. This is in contrast with caring for a mentally impaired person of any age which can sometimes involve continuous surveillance. Despite these factors there were issues which were, perhaps, unique to those caring for a spouse and which constrained the carers' ability to take time off.

Leaving the spouse unattended during the day

Just over half of the carers said that it was normally possible for them to leave their spouse alone for more than a few hours. However, for some this was possible only because there were other people around who were near enough to come over if the spouse needed anything. The other carers said that it was not possible for their spouse to be left alone for more than a few hours.

Mr Uckfield did actually leave his wife in order to go to work, but was able to do this only because he had relatives living with him and nearby who could come in to care for Mrs Uckfield. Until these relatives had arrived Mr Uckfield had regularly lost time from work. The others had little in the way of support and were very restricted in the amount of time they could spend away from home: 'You can't really leave [husband] on his own for long, you're sort of always, if you're going shopping you're on pins, if you like, has he fallen out of the chair?' (Mrs Ord, carer).

Going out, even if only for a couple of hours, involved many carers in extra worry and extra work preparing things so that the spouse could manage while alone. The decision to go out for the day, or even part of the day had to be taken very carefully, with due consideration for the spouse's current state of health. This was important not only because the spouse might not be able to cope that day, but also because the carers knew that they would not be able to relax if this was at the back of their minds.

For some carers the thought that their spouse was *alone*, rather than just without someone to give them help, clearly influenced the amount of time they were prepared to spend away. It was not too bad if they knew that the spouse had something with which to occupy his or her time:

> I knew he was all right to leave and he'd got a drawing that he were doing, a picture, so I knew more or less that he'd be sat drawing. The only thing he'd do would be mash a cup of tea or go to toilet and I knew he'd be all right else I wouldn't have gone. (Mrs Derby, carer)

If this was not the case then carers felt under some obligation to be with the spouse to provide companionship.

When spouses did not have activities they could pursue independently, carers felt themselves to be more restricted in the amount of time they could spend away. This could be the case even if the spouse was physically able to be left for more than a few hours. This is a slightly paradoxical finding in that, as we saw in Chapter 6, being together most of the time was a source of stress for many couples. Obviously, there was a conflict between keeping company with spouses who had no alternative source of occupation and leading the sort of life which would keep the relationship interesting. As we shall see later in this chapter some carers also felt uneasy about going out and enjoying themselves when their spouse could not join them.

Being away overnight

It was even less likely that carers would be able or willing to leave their spouses overnight. Only two carers, both men caring for wives who were not very disabled, said that there would usually be no problem being away overnight. However, both had experienced times in the past when they had been unable to leave their spouse or could anticipate a time in the future when it would become impossible to do so.

When pressed to say what they would do if there was no option but to be away overnight, say in the case of a family emergency, a third of carers said that, while they would not normally leave their partner overnight, in the case of absolute necessity a member of the family or, in one case, friends would stand in for them.

The remaining carers felt unable or unwilling to leave their spouse overnight and had no one they could call upon to help them out if needed. In some cases it was clear that the spouse might not be harmed by being left for one night, but that the carer would have been extremely worried all the time that she or he was away. Mrs Derby, for example, *had* been away from home overnight while she herself had been in hospital, but she would never have chosen to do this under any other circumstances and was not happy to think that she might have to repeat the experience. Her adult son and daughter had kept an eye on Mr Derby and had helped him with meals. However, Mrs Derby spent a lot of her time in hospital worrying about what was going on at home.

Some spouses actually needed attention during the night on a regular basis and others needed it from time to time, when their condition was particularly bad. Carers whose spouses were in this category were reluctant to leave them overnight *in case* something happened:

> When I first started with [employer] I said to him, 'Look . . . I'll come and work for you but on one condition, no nights out. Kiddies are growing up and leaving home and I must be home every night to make sure wife's OK . . .'. (Mr Linton, carer)

For the carers whose partners needed attention every or most nights there was just no obvious alternative to the carer's presence, especially when the help needed was of an unpredictable or intimate nature. For example, Mr Clifton had to be helped in and out of bed several times a night when he needed to go to the toilet, Mr Ord had to be helped on to the toilet at least once a night, Mrs Jefferson had to be turned when her legs became too painful to bear. Neither carers nor spouses thought it appropriate that relatives or neighbours should help with tasks of this sort and none had any ready access to a service which could replace the carer's input overnight. Only Mr Jefferson had the option of being away overnight, while his wife was in respite care once a fortnight, but he rarely used this time for himself because he still felt he should visit his wife at the hospital on the nights she was away.

Getting a break

The carers who found it difficult to leave their partners for more than a few hours or who could not contemplate being away from home overnight were asked whether they ever managed to get a break.

There was one carer whose only time away from her husband was the couple of hours a week she went out to do her shopping. Her husband, Mr Selsdon, was the most severely impaired spouse in the study and she trusted to luck, the sides on his hospital bed and sometimes a neighbour popping in, to ensure that nothing untoward happened while she was out. In the past she had been offered a day centre place for Mr Selsdon, but had not taken this up. At first she had been unable to get Mr Selsdon out of the house because there was no ramp for his wheelchair and now felt that he was too disabled to attend the centre:

> he sleeps a lot of the time now, and then I would always be worried in case he started any fits when he was awake.

Similarly, she had been offered hospital-based respite care, but was reluctant to take up the offer in case Mr Selsdon came home in a worse condition than he had been in when he left, as he had after previous admissions to hospital.

Other carers did manage to get breaks, but for some this was for only a few hours a week:

> I go to the hairdressers usually on a Friday . . . I count that as my day off . . . It's half a day from ten o'clock in the morning to just over 12, but I am entirely on my own. I think I owe it to myself . . . (Mrs Keighley, carer)

However, even a few hours away could help both carer and spouse even if the break was actually work or visiting relatives: 'Sundays I'll sometimes pop off down to me Mum's just for a break and I may take little 'un with me. [Husband] usually just relaxes, has a day to himself if he can. But if he's bad I don't leave him anyway' (Mrs Gifford, carer).

Planned breaks were unusual; Mr Jefferson was the only carer who was guaranteed respite, but this brought costs with it. Mrs Jefferson enjoyed neither the day centre she visited twice a week (and which she sometimes did not attend at all) nor the younger disabled person's unit (YDU) she entered once a fortnight. She went because she felt guilty about the responsibility her husband carried, but this, in its turn, put emotional pressure on Mr Jefferson and he never really felt free of responsibility. However, despite all the problems it created, he felt that he would not have been able to cope without these breaks.

As we saw in Chapter 4, Mr Jefferson's experiences of the difficulties associated with an unsatisfactory quality of respite care was in interesting contrast to that of Mrs Ord. Mr Ord had entered a YDU to enable his wife to have a holiday, but had refused to return. Mrs Ord had given in quietly:

We thought the idea was good, it gave me a break, but he wouldn't go back again because he was treated as a half-wit . . . So I can't really blame him for not wanting to go back.

These differences in outcome, in not dissimilar circumstances, seem to have their basis in differences in gender. At its baldest Mr Ord's interests came before those of Mrs Ord's and Mr Jefferson's before those of Mrs Jefferson's. The socialization processes that make it difficult for women to put their needs first are well documented. It is hardly surprising to find them at work in at least some of this group of married women.

However, there was another factor at work here; the nature of Mrs Jefferson's and Mr Ord's impairments. While both were similarly impaired physically – both used wheelchairs and needed similar types of help with personal care tasks – Mrs Jefferson's personality had undergone some change, apparently due to brain damage associated with her multiple sclerosis. The intermittently aggressive and inconsequential speech that were becoming more and more a part of Mrs Jefferson's behaviour made Mr Jefferson's job as a carer more difficult. However, it seemed that this change in personality also made it slightly easier for him to distance himself from Mrs Jefferson's dislike of the respite care facilities. This, in its turn, made it possible for him to continue using the service. By contrast, Mr Ord was the same person that Mrs Ord had married. This, combined with the reluctance to put her needs first, made it impossible for her to encourage Mr Ord to return to the YDU.

Under normal circumstances getting a break can come as much from going away *with* one's family or friends as it can from getting away *from* them. For some of the carers who had managed to go away from home with their spouses, however, it was often harder work than staying at home.

I'd rather not go [to parent's] to be perfectly honest with you. Like me Dad says, 'Now you can just do what you want when you come here' but you can't . . .

Really I prefer to stay at home. I'm more relaxed at home because [husband] can do what he wants and gets up when he wants and it doesn't matter how many times he gets up during the night, he's not disturbing anybody, only me. And he can make as many drinks as he wants and put telly on when he wants. (Mrs Clifton, carer)

Despite this some carers persevered with going away with their spouse (and family). Sometimes this was in order to keep in contact with their wider families, sometimes to maintain a sense of a normal life for their children, and sometimes because, despite everything, getting away was 'something to look forward to'.

I can see us just getting a break [this year] but a few weeks ago when he were dragging his leg about, I couldn't. I thought, oh flip; and you see *I* need a break more than anything. This is why [husband's] pushing it 'cos he says, this is what keeps me going an' all. I need something different, you know, just to keep me going 'cos with me having a lot to do and 'cos baby needs break 'cos she copes with it well, so it's a bit of morale for her really. Just need it. (Mrs Gifford, carer)

you've got to have something to look forward to and as far as doctor's concerned is, try and get breaks, as many breaks as you can – something to look forward to 'cos you can really get down. (Mrs Keighley, carer)

With this body

Social life

It was not surprising to find that many carers had experienced changes in their social life. This, also, is a finding paralleled in other studies of those caring for disabled people (Glendinning 1983; Baldwin 1985; Lewis and Meredith 1988).

For couples in this study, the loss of joint activities that had previously been an important part of the couples' lives together, was common:

> at one time we were never in. We wouldn't think anything of, when I finished work on a Friday night and he finished work on a Friday night, just come in, got a shower, pack the suitcase and off to . . . go to friends for the weekend, or a weekend down in . . . come back on the Sunday night, get ready to go to work the following morning. Well all that had to stop because he couldn't do it. (Mrs Ibstock, carer)

These reductions in social activity were not always the result solely of the physical aspects of the spouse's disability. Even when spouses were very severely disabled, lack of money could be more restrictive:

> if the financial situation was a little bit better it would certainly help . . .
> We could perhaps have better holidays, maybe afford to go out and have a meal more often, go out and have a drink more often . . . [or] go to the theatre or go anywhere. (Mr Jefferson, carer)

The loss of joint activities was particularly important for those carers who had not previously had an independent social life, because they lost their social life just as surely as their spouses had:

> we were always together, we've always been together, you know, I said we were like Torville and Dean. But sometimes over here the women [where wife works] have a night, they go somewhere for a night out . . . but trying to get her to go!
> *Interviewer: Won't she go?*
> Sometimes she will, but very rarely.
> *Interviewer: Why's that?*
> I don't know. I do know she doesn't like going thinking, 'well I'm here enjoying myself and he's sitting there' . . . (Mr Ibstock, spouse)

The difficulty of going out and having a good time without their spouse was implicit in several carers' accounts of why they preferred not to leave their partners for too long. Companionship was one of the supposed benefits of marriage, therefore, going away and leaving one's spouse alone was not really fair. This feeling was made most explicit by Mr Jefferson who used the language of adultery to describe how he sometimes felt when he took time for his own activities when his wife was in respite care:

> there would be absolute, goodness know *what* carry on if I went to the swimming baths and [wife] knew about it . . . so I had to give that sort of thing up except if I have me couple of days off I can do that and it's not that I'm being cheating, put it that way, I just go to the baths, have a good swim around, talk to some of the people I know. (Mr Jefferson, carer)

Although some spouses might be all right if left this did not always mean that the carer could continue with her or his social activities because other aspects of their lives left little time. Mr Eden had given up going to football matches when he was still working because he needed Saturday afternoons to do the housework and Mrs Gifford had given up a keep-fit class because: 'I haven't time to give Wednesday mornings up because if he's off [work] he needs me at home. And then when he's at work, I've usually got that much on, I usually catch up with things. So I just haven't time.'

In the absence of joint or single social activities, simple things could become very important for carers: 'Quite often [we] take the bus to [nearby town] . . . and get a taxi home . . . I buy as much as I possibly can [groceries] and it's an outing for the both of us – it's not very exciting but it's an outing' (Mrs Keighley, carer).

Those couples who had managed to keep a car (see Chapter 7) were clearly better off in regard to getting out and could enjoy some activities together from time to time, even if it was only driving to the nearest beach and looking at the sea. When cars had been given up, either because the carer could not drive or for financial reasons, even these small pleasures became well nigh impossible:

Interviewer: Do you regret not being able to drive?
Oh yes, I do. It's the biggest regret that I ever had because in that way, well I could have managed the two of us, you know, I could have managed to take him out. (Mrs Keighley, carer)

A few carers did manage to maintain some form of independent social life, particularly through church activities (see Chapter 3), but they were in the minority and were caring for spouses whose needs for help were not usually great during the day.

Finding time to be ill

Having time off from caring is not just about elective social and leisure activities, of course. Carers, like anyone else, get ill and need time to recuperate. Because of the lack of alternative sources of help, finding time to be ill was particularly problematic for this group, despite the fact that some of them had substantial health problems of their own. Questions about what would happen if the carer were to be ill underlined just how vulnerable and unsupported some of the couples in this study were.

Just over half of the carers said that their family (usually grown children), friends or neighbours would help them out if necessary, but it was clear that this help would be suitable only for fairly short-term crises. For most the prospect of being ill for more than a day or so was a source of great anxiety:

Interviewer: What do you think would happen if you ever were ill?
Oh I dread to think. I do, I dread to think. That's just something I don't think about if I can help it because I don't know what he'd do. (Mrs Baker, carer)

Carrying on although ill was a common occurrence among carers and, as we saw in Chapter 4, carers who had been in hospital themselves often failed to get the convalescence that they needed. Other carers who had been quite seriously ill had delayed going to their doctor because they were worried about the possibility of going into hospital or had resisted going into hospital at all. Mrs Ibstock, for example, had seen a specialist who suspected that she had appendicitis. He had wanted to admit her to hospital immediately, but she had persuaded him to let her go home and 'get things worked out'. Her condition had turned out to be far more serious than originally suspected: '[the specialist] said for appendix I would only be in for two days. Well when they had to do that big operation I was worrying myself sick and they kept us in for 14 days before they would let us home . . .' (Mrs Ibstock, carer).

The carers' sensation of being on their own was most acute when they were ill. Even if they were able to take to their beds few could expect even the occasional cup of tea, although some spouses would struggle to do what they could to help. When in hospital carers spent the empty hours worrying about their spouses, and even though they were keen to get home they knew that there was little hope of a few days of taking it easy and being cared for :

> so [after coming out of hospital] it was only a matter of cooking but I mean I felt that weak I didn't even have energy to cook, I felt . . . well, you know what it is, after an operation you've kind of got to have some time. Well for two mornings I were able to stay in bed and [husband] brought me a cup of tea but I know what a trial it is to him doing it so I *have* to get up, he is willing enough but by the time he gets to top of stairs then he has to sit down. (Mrs Derby, carer)

Formal support to carers and spouses was minimal, even when carers were quite ill themselves, and carers' own medical needs were overlooked by professionals close to the situation. With no ready access to supportive services it was illness of the carer that seemed, in the end, most likely to lead to breaks in the relationship.

Given the ages of carers in this study it was, perhaps, not so surprising to find a high level of ill-health among them. Fewer than a third said, unequivocally, that their health was good. Of the remainder, three had had major abdominal operations in the three years previous to the interview and four had arthritis and/or back complaints. Another seven suffered from a range of chronic problems; eczema and/or asthma, diabetes and a stomach ulcer, colitis, bronchitis, a kidney complaint and anaemia, and arterial sclerosis. There was also a carer who had recently had meningitis followed by clinical depression which recurred from time to time. As the figures indicate some carers had multiple health problems.

A few carers had complaints which, under normal circumstances, might have made *them* the disabled partner in the couple; it was only a matter of history that they were not. Their spouse had been injured or ill first and, therefore, they had taken on the carer role. Mrs Keighley, for example, had a kidney complaint, which caused her considerable distress. She was on permanent medication and her husband said that she also had a chronic form of anaemia for which she received 'liver injections'. Mr Eden had adult onset diabetes and a stomach ulcer, and had been away from work for over a year at the time of the interview. Mrs Ord had developed colitis some ten months before being interviewed, and during its acute phase had lost one and a half stone in weight.

Unsupported caring could also take its toll psychologically. Seven carers, two of them men, reported that they were often stressed or suffered from 'nerves', conditions which they saw as directly related to the responsibilities which they carried and which often affected their physical health: 'I had a spell like this [with rapid heart beat] before Christmas, this was when I were trying to cope with everything and I think it got a bit too much and [the doctor] put me tablets up to an extra one' (Mrs Clifton, carer). All the carers who reported symptoms of this sort had spouses who were amongst the most disabled.

None of the carers who had serious conditions and few of those with more minor complaints were likely to improve much in the future, not least because many of them were in their late forties or fifties and had conditions, such as arthritis, which were degenerative. Anxieties about their ability to carry on, especially among those who realized that the stresses and strains of caring made things worse, were very real: 'God willing I keep my health for as long as I can but there will come a time [when] I can't or even if I die she'll have to go in [to residential care]' (Mr Jefferson, carer).

Finally, it is worth drawing attention again to the problems that some carers had had in getting their own health needs recognized. Both Mrs Derby and Mrs Ibstock had returned home after major abdominal surgery with instructions not to lift anything or do heavy housework. Neither had been able to keep to these instructions and Mrs Derby had severe internal bleeding soon after returning home. Mrs Ord had been left totally unsupported at home with cracked and bruised ribs, and a husband who needed lifting in and out of the bath, and up and downstairs. Mr Quincy was sent home from hospital after his attack of meningitis, still vomiting and unsteady on his feet, to a wife with arthritis of the spine and hip, and who was prone to depression. Early discharge policies in hospitals and the lack of proper support services in the community imposed costs on these women and men that are hardly defensible in the late twentieth century:

> the last night I was in [hospital] all I could think of really was, I wished I could have another couple of days because I knew that I was going to come home and have to start and I knew that I couldn't really muster it up. But we got through. (Mrs Derby, carer)

The experience of caring for a spouse

The whole of this book has, of course, in some sense been about the experience of caring for a disabled spouse. However, we have tended to concentrate on the specific effects of caring and disability rather than on what it is *like* to care for one's spouse. In this section of the chapter we turn to concentrate on what carers said about the experience of caring – about the difficulties it presented, about the effect it had on them as people, about how it actually felt to provide help, over and above that normally expected, to the man or woman they had married.

Being a 'professional'

During the interviews we talked to carers about how, if at all, helping a husband or wife was different from helping, say, a child or parent. There was a subgroup of carers, all women, who had either cared for other kin in the past or who had current responsibilities. Two had very extensive past caring histories. Mrs Baker had cared for both her father and father-in-law, who had lived with the couple, when her children were young. Before that she had nursed her mother until her death. Mrs Fowey had looked after her mother-in-law and, after she became ill and died, her father-in-law.

This intensive involvement made it apparently more difficult for these carers to see any difference between what they did then for others and what they did now for their husbands. They were well and truly professional carers (cf. Ungerson 1987) and the fact that they were now caring for a husband was more or less incidental:

> it makes no difference. I've looked after umpteen.
> *Interviewer: Do you think it's any different [caring for a husband]?*
> No. I think because, if they're poorly, they need some sort of help, don't they? They need some sort of help, they need attention. (Mrs Fowey, carer)

By contrast, some of the women who had current responsibilities for the care of others were able to see differences in the experience. Mrs Ibstock, for example, did her mother's shopping and went round to see her most days. When her mother was 'bad' she had to help her into bed at night, get her up in the morning and cook for her. However, she felt that this was easier than caring for her husband because, if she had to help her mother with personal care, her *mother* would have been less embarrassed than was her husband:

> when a woman's got to look after a woman in that way for baths it's not as bad 'cos she's a woman but I think when a wife's got to do it for her husband I think it's degrading on the husband's part to think that his wife's got to come to that, to bathing, drying and powdering and wash his head. (Mrs Ibstock, carer)

We dealt with the issue of 'cross-sex caring' in Chapter 2; here its importance seems to lie in the fact that Mrs Baker and Mrs Fowey had provided close personal care for men in the past (both father and father-in-law) and, therefore, had got over a barrier which other carers had not. They had, perhaps, gone through some process akin to that which formal carers, such as nurses, go through when they start to provide intimate care. Other carers' experiences also suggest this. Mrs Mead, for example, when talking about the personal care her husband had needed when he came out of hospital said: 'Well, as I say, with me being a home help, I'd done all that so it was OK, it was more embarrassing for him than me . . .'.

Sometimes, however, the 'professionalization' of the spouse carer's role could go too far:

> there are . . . some terrific problems. Where do you, for instance, where do you, when do you stop being a nurse and become a husband? And when there is an almost continual demand upon you . . . but I sometimes feel, oh I just work here, that sort of thing. (Mr Jefferson, carer)

And, of course, in the final analysis the informal carer was *not* a professional because, as Mr Jefferson pointed out, the carer could not leave the job behind at the end of the working day: '. . . the doctors, nurses, social workers, whatever, you do have – if you do your job you can go away from it' (Mr Jefferson, carer).

'You feel it more inside'

Not all carers were able to talk about how, if at all, caring for a spouse might be different from caring for other relatives, particularly if they had had no other experience of caring (cf. Ungerson 1987). Others, however, were very clear both that there were differences and about where these differences lay.

First, there was the challenge to normal expectations which caring for a disabled spouse presented:

> When it's your parents [you are caring for] . . . well it's different. You take it in your stride more. You expect it, you don't expect it but you know that it happens. People that are older and need help and sympathy, whatever, that's a different kind of thing altogether. When it's your partner, well you're both of an age more or less and it's harder to take. (Mrs Keighley, carer)

These challenged expectations were closely related to the nature of what one had to do as a spouse carer:

> when you're doing it for a man it's more embarrassing than anything. With a child, you know, it's what you're *supposed* to do for a child and that, it is very embarrassing, especially your own husband. I mean with a stranger, you know, but with your husband it is very embarrassing.
> *Interviewer: Even though he is your husband?*
> Yes. I mean I'd never seen him in that way before, lying there, not being able to do anything and with embarrassment . . . it used to make him very bad tempered. (Mrs Mead, carer)

Furthermore, as both Mrs Keighley's and Mrs Mead's words suggest, the temporary loss of adult status that the spouse experienced while being cared for caused problems for both carers and spouses.

Secondly, caring for a spouse was different because it hurt the carer more to see the spouse in pain or restricted in his or her life:

> You could help [others] but, you could help and it wouldn't hurt you so much. You'd feel happy that you were able to help and that would be it. It wouldn't hurt you. (Mrs Keighley, carer)

> although I love me parents and I love me children, I love me wife, I find it harder to care for her than the children or me parents. I don't know *why* actually. I mean it upsets me when the children are ill . . . I don't know really, I suppose I *am* more concerned about [wife] when she's ill than me children . . . (Mr Quincy, carer)

It seemed to be more difficult for these carers to distance themselves emotionally from their spouses than it would have been to do so from other kin, even – for some it seemed – their children. This is not totally surprising because being close emotionally is, at least as conventionally portrayed, the main *raison d'être* of marriage. Thus, while we love our children because they are our children and love our parents because they are our parents, by contrast our spouses are our spouses because we love them. Consequently, even if we stop loving our parents or children they remain, nonetheless, our parents and children. If we no longer love our spouses one of the main reasons for *being* a spouse is removed.

Ungerson (1987) has pointed to the extent to which people caring *for* their parents 'found it easier to forget about caring *about* them, since some of their emotions were too distressing' (p. 116). This is not an option open to spouse carers unless they undermine the very basis of their relationship or, alternatively, change the nature of it.

Various commentators have suggested that if the nature of the relationship does change carers are most likely to adopt a mothering model of care; in the case of spouse carers reconstructing their husbands as children (Ungerson 1987; Borsay 1990). In this sample of younger spouse carers there was only one carer (a woman) who had obviously adopted the mothering role in order to help her to cope and her husband was in no physical or mental condition to challenge this. By contrast, most other spouses resisted to varying degrees any attempt to cast them into the role of quasi-children and carers were mostly very aware of the distress which the help they provided to their spouses caused them. These carers, thus, had no alternative model of care-giving which they could adopt to reduce stress. They were married to partners who, for the most part, they still loved; if those partners were in pain or were distressed the carers shared in that pain and distress.

The third difference which carers pointed to was the combination of physical and emotional closeness which helping a spouse necessarily entailed. Caring for a parent usually takes place somewhere else and one can walk away from it (Parker and Lawton 1992); caring for a spouse was inevitably done in the same household. Even caring for a severely disabled child would involve time apart while the child attended school and elderly disabled people in the same household might go to a day centre or similar. By contrast, the combination of co-residence and the lack of any acceptable, alternative daytime activity for the spouse meant that close and almost continuous contact was the norm (Oliver 1983; and see Chapter 6). When combined with the provision of substantial personal care, this could become very destructive:

> you've done all this and then there's yet another demand. You say, oh I feel like a robot, a machine – not all the time, sometimes. It's far too close an environment to be in, it is not good for the disabled person and it's not good for the carer. (Mr Jefferson, carer)

The final major difference about caring for a spouse mentioned by carers was that when one cared for a spouse there was no one else to share that job with, and that one had to take on the spouse's job as well. This was particularly problematic if there were young children to be cared for.

Change

Life had changed in many ways for most of the couples in the study, but some carers felt that the experience of caring had changed them very fundamentally, both as people and in relation to the role or niche which they occupied in their community or in society in general. Carers who were fairly young when their spouses had become disabled and/or those whose spouses had been affected suddenly spoke most often about these changes. The reason for this latter effect is obvious; the former seems to be associated with the extent to which couples saw themselves as different from their peers. Carers who were older at onset of the spouse's disability shared the experience of their spouse's failing health or increasing impairment with at least some of their contemporaries; this was very rarely the case for those who were young.

The major change which female carers spoke about was to do with becoming more independent or self-reliant and taking on more responsibility. For some, like Mrs Derby and Mrs Keighley, taking on additional responsibilities, particularly for financial matters and decision making, had been a relatively temporary phenomenon, while their husbands had been particularly ill. For others the changes were more permanent and in some circumstances, carers felt, not all bad: 'when we first got married [husband] . . . dealt with all the money. Now we both do it, so we both know where it's going . . . it's better that it is shared' (Mrs Ord, carer).

Carers also felt that they were changed people:

> I am definitely different. I probably am a bit harder because you have to be more independent, you have to stick up for yourself a bit more and get it done. I know I've changed, definitely. I mean I'm not that hard, don't get me wrong, but like I say, you've just got to adjust yourself to it and be determined. Got to have a lot of that, definitely. (Mrs Gifford, carer)

Their ability to take on extra responsibilities and to undertake new things often surprised them: 'If anybody had told me before I got married that I'd be doing this, I would have said, no way, I couldn't cope with it. But I suppose it's always surprising what you can do when you *have* to do it' (Mrs Ord, carer).

One might have expected that the areas in which changed responsibilities would be problematic for carers would be where they challenged normal gender roles in the household. Interestingly, such changes were not necessarily a problem for the carers personally, but they were often aware that others, outside the household, might consider their behaviour unusual. This was the same for both men and women:

> I'm noted for going up and down with barrow. But, and then they [neighbours] think, 'God, she's doing it and he in't' but it's just some'at – I just do. (Mrs Gifford, carer)

> there are certain things that it's sort of OK for women to do and is a little bit frowned upon if a man does it, like hanging the washing out. *I* don't *mind* doing that at all but there are people that think, you know, they come out with [remarks] like, 'You'll make somebody a good wife', which is a bit snide and a bit nasty but somebody has to do it so therefore in the end I say well, I'll have to do it. (Mr Jefferson, carer)

Similarly, spouses' feelings that carers were having to take on jobs that were 'by right' their (the spouses') responsibility could also make carers feel that they were transgressing boundaries:

> one particular time I had the washer on and I went upstairs and she were crying 'cos I had to do washing and it were a novelty to me, you know. I said, 'It don't matter', you know, I don't mind washing. (Mr Picton, carer)

There were carers who felt that role change was difficult to cope with although, as in Mrs Ibstock's case, this appeared to be as much to do with having to do *everything* as it was with having to do jobs not normally associated with being a woman:

> when I've got a great big cutter . . . and I'm standing out there and I'm cutting the privet . . . I'm saying, I shouldn't be doing this, it's not my job, this is a man's job and I'm digging, putting apple trees in the garden and I'm saying it's not my job. But it's what you've got to do, so you just get on with it.

The third main aspect of change which carers felt in themselves was their separateness; like a rite of passage the experience of caring had in some sense set them apart from the uninitiated. Consequently, 'nobody else could understand' what caring was like:

> there's all kind of problems crop up that you wouldn't, you couldn't think of if you weren't living with a person that's disabled . . .
>
>   Anybody that deals with, whose partner is disabled, they wouldn't think the same way as a person who doesn't have to deal with this everyday. They can't possibly.
> (Mrs Keighley, carer)

While these feelings of separateness or difference could help carers to value themselves (see Chapter 6) they could also, of course, cut them off from a sense of belonging and the emotional support that might come with it:

> It does get me down occasionally but it's a case of, there's not many people you can talk to about it. I go down and talk to me Dad about it and that's all really, 'cos there's not many people understand what you have to put up with . . . (Mrs Gifford, carer)

Conclusions

This chapter has attempted to describe the nature of caring for a spouse, pointing particularly to the areas in which the experiences of spouse carers seemed to be similar to or different from those of other carers.

Like many others, spouse carers felt unable to leave the cared-for person for long periods. However, in the almost total absence of services, unless there was someone else living in or nearby the home who could substitute for the carer, spouse carers were particularly limited in their ability to get out at any time. In this respect they have more in common with single carers than they do with, say, married couples caring for a disabled child or an elderly relative. The lack of alternative day-time activities for the spouse tied carers even more securely to the home.

The inability or unwillingness of carers to leave the home meant that their own social lives were curtailed and many had also lost joint activities that had previously been an important part of their married lives. However, joint social activities were affected not only by the physical environment, but also by financial considerations; even if they had been able to get out some couples could not have afforded to do so.

The relatively isolated position which spouse carers occupied was highlighted by their attitudes to their own ill health. Many felt that they could not afford to be ill and, if they ever were, played down their symptoms or took less time to recover than they might otherwise have done. There was a lot of physical ill-health and mental stress, particularly amongst the most involved carers, some of it apparently related to carrying caring responsibilities. There were some frankly appalling gaps in the provision of health care for carers, particularly when they returned home from hospital. Given that many of the conditions carers suffered from were degenerative, and given the fact that many of them were in or approaching middle-age, it was clear that they would become increasingly vulnerable in the future.

A few carers, particularly those who had previous caring responsibilities, appeared to take the whole experience in their stride. The majority, however, found it distressing. Becoming a carer had challenged their expectations about the form their lives would take. The closeness of their relationship with their partner made their experience more painful, they felt, than if they had been caring for some other member of the family. Like single carers for older people they had no one else with whom to share either the physical or the emotional responsibilities of caring. Unlike single carers, the nature of their relationship with their spouse made it difficult, if not impossible, for them to distance themselves from the experience.

Finally, the interviews demonstrated that caring for a spouse distanced respondents psychologically from their peers. Their experiences appeared almost like a rite of passage. While this could be, for some, a psychologically helpful feeling, allowing them to see themselves as exceptional, it also had the effect of making it difficult for them to share their experiences. Other people, they felt, 'did not really understand' and could, therefore, provide little in the way of emotional support.

One of the most striking things to emerge from this chapter is, perhaps, how like other carers spouses are in many respects. They experience similar restrictions in their ability to get out and to have a social life as do other carers. Like other carers they feel that they cannot afford to be ill, and they find cross-sex caring just as difficult as do people who are not married to one another.

This similarity is particularly important because, as Oliver (1983) has argued, there is a tendency for service provision to be built around 'the assumption that the ability to cope is bestowed with the wedding ring' (p. 73). This research has shown that spouse carers are no more or less likely to cope than anyone else and that marriage does not magically endow spouse carers with personality characteristics that make it easier for them than for anyone else.

However, the similarity with other carers is not complete. The nature of the emotional relationship implied by the ideal of modern marriage – close, companionate, joint, 'equal' (even if the partners' roles are different) – adds to the felt impact of caring when a partner is involved. Spouse carers are unable to distance themselves from those they are caring for or to adopt alternative models of caring (such as the mothering model) which might help them cope psychologically. Consequently, caring can hurt a lot emotionally.

Both the similarities and the differences point to the necessity to provide support for younger disabled people and their carers. Their needs are certainly no less and in some instances may be much greater than other groups.

Conclusions

As argued in the introductory chapter, the absence of marriage from the debate on community care, whether that debate has been led by feminist scholars or by the disabled people's movement, has led to some serious gaps in our knowledge about and understanding of disability and caring. Its inclusion and integration into these debates can, I believe, help us forward. Also in the first chapter, a number of areas in which these gaps led to particular misunderstandings were outlined. What has the evidence presented throughout the book contributed to increased understanding of these?

Marriage makes it easier

We have seen that marriage does not make the experience of disability and caring easier. To use Judith Oliver's (1983) phrase again, the ability to cope is not magically 'bestowed with the wedding ring'. Younger married couples seem to find themselves in a particularly disadvantaged position. They are badly served by formal services which would support the disabled partner, leaving the carer to provide the bulk of personal and physical help that is required. Consequently, if disabled men leave paid work their wives, both because of their unequal position in the labour market and because they have to help and support their husbands, are unable fully to replace the men's earnings. The husbands of disabled women, because of the nature of the labour market for men, especially for those in manual occupations, are unlikely to be able to sustain any paid work if helping their wives beyond a certain level. Unlike in many other situations (in particular where offspring are caring for older parents in the same household or where disabled children are being cared for) there is no one else in the household to provide at least one main earner's wage. The younger the couple are when the spouse becomes disabled, the worse their situation is. The presence of young children adds further to couples' difficulties.

Few couples have informal networks which *could* help the disabled spouse; but in any case such a potential source of help is seen to be inappropriate. Furthermore, because of the lack of help generally, younger couples are prevented from forging neighbourhood and friendship networks which might support them in other, more appropriate, ways.

Providing intimate personal care to a spouse is *not* made easier by marriage; indeed, it may be made more difficult because it can constrain a couple's sexual relationship in both subtle and not so subtle ways. Additional strain can be added to the relationship when the spouse's impairments are such that a sexual relationship is difficult or impossible.

Disabled women, male carers

The evidence of this study adds support to the growing recognition that women can be *more* disabled than men in comparable circumstances. If they remain in the labour market, as women they have lower incomes anyway. If they are not in the labour market, indirect discrimination in the state benefits system means that they are likely to receive lower levels of benefits. Their need for help and support may be seen as less important, and their desire to retain control over domestic arrangements may be over-ridden by the provision of services which serve to replace, rather than enable, their role.

Women who become disabled after marriage are also affected by the pre-existing dynamics of the relationship. In marriages where power is particularly unequal, disabled women may find themselves very constrained in their ability to assert their needs. Even where power is not so unequal, women's general reluctance to assert their needs before those of other family members may find disabled women doing things they would rather not (like entering respite care) or not doing things that they would rather (for example, retaining control over domestic arrangements).

Husbands who help and support disabled wives thus find themselves in a somewhat paradoxical position. On the one hand, if not in paid work they share in their disabled wives' poverty and have to compensate for the lack of recognition of her needs by service providers. On the other hand, they may benefit (in comparison to women caring for disabled husbands) from their greater power in the relationship and from their wives' unwillingness to assert their needs.

This is not to argue that disabled men are in any particularly advantaged position – the evidence presented in this book could hardly support such a view – but rather to point up more clearly the extra disadvantage that disabled women (and to some degree their husbands) experience.

This book has also contributed something to our understanding of how men experience care-giving and why, within marriage at least, they do it. As we have seen, many of the differences between male and female spouses, and between male and female carers have their basis in structural inequalities between men and women, and differences in gender roles. However, husbands' and wives' *feelings* about care-giving and their reasons for continuing with it were more alike than previous analysis would have predicted. Men, in similar proportions to women, referred to ideas of duty or reciprocity in talking about why they continued to help and support their partners. Men as well as women provided intimate personal care when it was needed and both sexes found it difficult, at least initially, partly because their spouses found it difficult too.

With this body

Whether or not these similarities are due to the fact that people were *married* remains to be tested. What is clear is that men have to be incorporated into future research and analysis of informal care.

Both sides of the coin

This cross-cutting of the generalized disadvantage experienced by all disabled people with the particular disadvantage experienced by women (or black people or older people) is one of the major issues to emerge when both sides of the disability/caring relationship are explored. It lends an inevitable complexity to a picture that has previously been presented in a rather simple fashion.

One aspect of that complexity which emerges from this study was the way in which couples negotiated the spouse's independence and its presentation to the rest of the world. This meant that there was a process of negotiation both within the relationship itself, and between the couple and others.

Spouses and carers had to come to some agreement about the extent to which the spouse would do things for him/herself. Sometimes this meant that extra work or anxiety was created for the carer. If the disabled partner had access to paid help which he or she could direct, any such cost would, in theory, be compensated for by pay. In the absence of paid help, however, carers were sometimes keen to reduce or prevent these costs to themselves and, thus, imposed costs on their partner. Others were prepared to bear the extra costs because they knew how important it was to the spouse to remain as independent as possible.

The couples also negotiated the spouse's independence with people outside the relationship. For some this meant preventing knowledge about the spouse's need for help with everyday tasks spreading much beyond the couple themselves. As a consequence, help from outside the relationship, even that offered from formal sources, might be refused by the spouse or by the carer. For these couples, then, there really did not seem to be an acceptable alternative to the carer's assistance with personal and physical care. This may be different from situations where marriage happens *after* one of the partners has become disabled, especially if he or she is already used to having someone other than a close family member provide support. In either situation, however, the presence of a third party to the relationship may offer a considerable challenge to conventional norms of married life. In criticizing some of the solutions to reliance on informal carers proposed by feminists (see below), Morris has pointed out that it is hardly fair to expect disabled people to be in the vanguard of the assault on conventional family forms (Morris 1991). The same surely applies to those attempting to preserve some degree of ordinariness in their marriage, especially when they live in communities where traditional forms are still very strong.

Seeing both sides also shows clearly that disabled people, and those who provide them with help and support on an unpaid basis have, or should have, a *common* agenda for change, albeit that certain elements of that agenda might be different for different groups of disabled people and their carers. We turn to that agenda now, in the final section of this chapter and of the book.

A common agenda?

Two contributions to a seminar held in London in 1990, entitled 'The needs and resources of disabled people', set out an agenda for disabled people and for carers. Richard Wood, Director of the British Council of Organisations of Disabled People, said in his contribution to the book based on the seminar:

> Let us state what disabled people do want by first stating what we don't want.
>
> WE DON'T WANT CARE!!!!
>
> To lead full and equal lives in the community, disabled people need:
>
> (a) Full access in every sense of the word. Not just access to the environment but full and equal access to education (including higher education), training, employment and information.
> (b) Transport systems which we can use on main routes on demand.
> (c) A programme for accessible housing to ensure that disabled people have full mobility within and between communities.
> (d) Access to the real technical aids which we need to assist us to achieve independence.
> (e) Personal support services which are directly under our own control, or that of a chosen advocate.
> (f) The right to choose where and how to live.
> (g) The right to equal opportunities and not just 'everything being equal' equal opportunities.
>
> (Wood 1991: 201–202)

In her contribution, Jill Pitkeathley, Director of Carers National Association, said that carers needed recognition, information, practical help, money and time off. She also stated that carers rarely say 'that they want *more* consideration, *more* help, *more* money than the person for whom they are caring. Rather, they almost inevitably take the view that the needs of both people must be considered together and separately in order to ensure a better deal for *both*' (Pitkeathley 1991: 203, original emphasis).

Against both of these proposed 'solutions' we can pose that developed by feminists, principally Finch (1984) and Dalley (1988). Their analysis sees women's responsibility for informal care as rooted in their conventional responsibilities for domestic service and child care. Responsibility for other forms of care, they argue, grows out of this. The solution, therefore, is to challenge and look for creative alternatives to family models of care.

Do these three positions, which seem so different, offer us any hope of movement forward?

Wood is arguing from the theoretical position which asserts that disability is socially created and that, therefore, social and economic change can prevent individuals with impairments becoming disabled. Leaving aside for a moment the issue of personal support, the achievement of his agenda would, indeed, reduce the numbers of people needing help and support from their family, friends or neighbours. The addition of the personal support item would totally remove the need for carers. There are, however, problems with Wood's agenda in its entirety, which centre around this issue of personal support. First, as we have seen, the provision of personal support services from outside is likely both to threaten certain sorts of relationships, particularly established marriages, and to run counter to what some disabled people within those relationships want. Secondly, his proposals ignore the fact that existing power dynamics will influence choice; some women, in particular, will remain the main providers of personal support services because that is what those whom they care for will wish. Thirdly, his agenda is primarily one for younger adults. The provision of personal care exclusively by others fits oddly against expectations of normal family life for severely impaired young children, for example.

Pitkeathley's agenda, although it acknowledges the needs of the disabled person, is about marginal improvement within the *status quo*. As we saw in the first chapter, carers have taken the high ground in recent years, mainly because they serve important policy (and political) purposes. The carers' lobby does not, however, challenge the social creation of disability and, therefore, of carers. Rather, it seeks to temper the experience of providing informal care by encouraging the visibility of carers and the development of services which meet their needs. Unlike Wood, Pitkeathley acknowledges that disability and caring take place within existing relationships, that the dynamics of these can be important, and that the needs of the disabled person and the carer may conflict.

The feminist solution to the question of informal care, as rehearsed by Dalley and Finch, is to challenge 'familism' and provide alternatives to family models of care. This challenge, however, is to *start* with disabled people and the alternatives are to be an enhanced quality of residential care or communal (collective) forms of living. Morris (1991) has pointed out that many disabled people have to fight hard to maintain any form of family life. To imply some form of 'false consciousness' because they wish to adopt conventional modes of family organization is, she claims, to add insult to injury. Others have also started to acknowledge that this essentially white, non-disabled, middle class critique fails other groups, for example black and working class women, and for similar reasons (Williams 1989; Graham 1991). Furthermore, as the creation of disability is not central to the analysis, solutions which might reduce disability, *per se*, are not seen as inextricably linked to the feminist design.

None of these positions offers a complete solution to the informal care issue, but the elements essential for progress are evident in all three.

The first step is to acknowledge that disability is socially created and that action committed to reducing the effects of a disabling social, economic and physical environment will also reduce the need for anyone, man or woman, to provide informal care. Within this commitment, however, there has to be a recognition that the existing dynamics of relationships and women's position within them would be unchanged. It also has to be recognized that different people – women, black people, older people, those who are ill as well as disabled – have their disability created in different ways. The agenda will not be the same for all, and neither will the way in which they wish to have their needs for personal support met.

That some people *will* wish to have their personal support needs met through informal relationships means that there will still be informal carers. A continuing feminist analysis is necessary to point out why, in many cases, it will still be women who become carers, but it must also start to incorporate the growing evidence about the involvement of men and how this can be encouraged (Baldwin and Twigg 1991). Furthermore, this analysis will also have to acknowledge the two-way exchange; 'the reciprocity involved in caring relationships and the threats to that reciprocity . . . because it is the loss of reciprocity which brings about inequality within a relationship – and disabled and older people are very vulnerable within the unequal relationships which they commonly experience with the non-disabled world' (Morris 1991: 163). As Morris goes on to point out, dependence on a partner or family member is exploitive to *both* sides if it is necessary because of a lack of any alternative.

Finally, because some people will continue to provide unpaid help and support – the parents of disabled children, some spouses, some offspring of mentally impaired older people – there will be a continued need for recognition of their contribution and support for *them* as well as for the person they help.

A P P E N D I X

Design, sampling, methods and characteristics of the couples

Method, design and sample

The sampling frame

The OPCS disablement survey of adults (Martin *et al.* 1988) was used as a sampling frame as it offered several advantages over any other method of sample selection. First, the survey was large (around 8,000 achieved interviews) and designed to over-represent younger people. Secondly, the survey was nationally based, offering the opportunity to cluster interviews regionally. Thirdly, a series of questions in the survey established the level of help with self-care activities that the person who was disabled needed and received. Answers to these and other questions could be used to determine whether or not the respondent's spouse was his/her main carer. Finally, respondents to the OPCS survey had been asked at the time they were interviewed whether they would have any objection to being followed-up by researchers at some point in the future.

The focus of the study and nature of the sample to be sought

Beyond the decision to focus on the experience of younger couples other considerations influenced the nature of the sample. The most important of these was to include only spouses whose disability had become apparent *after* marriage in order to concentrate on changes that may happen to married couples when one of them becomes disabled and their previous expectations about their life together are disrupted.

By doing this the potential sample was limited in two further ways. First, a range of congenital conditions, such as cerebral palsy, muscular dystrophy and spina bifida, were excluded. Conditions with a genetic *cause*, but which do not manifest themselves until adulthood, e.g. Huntington's chorea, were not necessarily excluded by this. Secondly, the length of time for which the spouse had been disabled was, by definition, limited by the duration of the marriage.

The second decision about the nature of the sample was to limit it to spouses who said that they needed some help with self-care from another person, at least once or twice a day and/or at any time during the night. Those who did not require much help with self-care, but who needed someone to be with them most of the time in order to avoid danger to themselves were also included.

Finally, no spouses whose *primary* disabling condition was a mental health problem were included in the study. This did not, however, exclude the possibility of a spouse who had mental health problems *in addition* to a physical impairment being included in the sample.

Rationale for a qualitative approach

Both marriage and disablement are complex social phenomena and potentially sensitive topics for a research project; thorough investigation of either needs time and has the potential for generating extremely rich data. A quantitative approach would inevitably have constrained the extent to which this complexity and richness could be drawn out and might have imposed on it a structure which did not tally with respondents' own experiences and views. The younger people identified through the OPCS disablement survey constituted a precious sample uncontaminated by service receipt, membership of a self-help organization or some other identifying variable. By definition, they provided access to information about the widest possible range of experiences and needs. To constrain this group by imposing a quasi-experimental design, or by attempting to define it so that it would become acceptable within a quantitative mode of research, would have been to waste much of the variety within it and the knowledge that could be gained from that variety.

All this pointed to an approach which could cope with, indeed welcomed, variability in a small group of respondents. The grounded theory approach, originally outlined by Glaser and Strauss (1967), and subsequently used successfully in both pure and applied fields (Walker 1985), appeared to offer this.

Carrying out the project

Sample selection

OPCS identified 67 potential respondents who met the criteria for inclusion in the sampling frame. That is, they were: under retirement age; married, with a spouse also under retirement age; had an impairment which was not congenital or of childhood onset and which had started since marriage; needed an amount of care over the threshold set for the study; and had said that they were willing to be re-interviewed. In addition, respondents were restricted to those living in the North of England.

By the time sampling actually took place the 67 potential respondents had been reduced by 17 due to an RNIB study of people with impaired vision which had also used respondents from the OPCS survey.

Contacting the potential respondents and response rate

For reasons of confidentiality OPCS made the initial contacts with the 50 potential respondents, four of whom were proxies (i.e. people who had responded on the disabled person's behalf). Of these, eleven told OPCS that they did not wish to take part in the spouse carer survey, one respondent had died, and two had moved away and were unable to be contacted. Of the 36 contacts eventually supplied by OPCS three were proxies.

OPCS provided names, addresses and, where available, telephone numbers. Where telephone numbers were provided the researcher attempted to make direct contact with potential respondents to gather a small amount of preliminary information to help guide the pattern of selection and interviewing, and to establish the practicality of carrying out separate interviews with the spouses. Where telephone numbers were not available, or had changed and could not be updated, a letter and short questionnaire were sent out.

The additional contact prompted further refusals (four). In addition, another potential respondent was found to have died, one had returned to his home country and five did not respond to further communication. One respondent had separated from his wife, who was still living in the marital home; and the wife was retained in the pool of respondents. The achieved pool of respondents was thus 25 (a response rate of 74 per cent of 34 achievable contacts). Further attempts at communication with the five non-responders were unsuccessful.

Twenty couples and two carers were eventually interviewed (a total of 42 interviews). One spouse was unable to participate and one had left the marital home. The other three couples who had agreed to be interviewed eventually withdrew from the project, in two cases because one partner had agreed to participate without consulting the other, who had then refused.

The information which was gathered about the couples in the initial contact was used to determine the order in which interviews were carried out. It was decided to start with the most typical couples; those aged 50 or over, with no dependent children at home, and where the spouse had a gradually deteriorating condition which had been present for ten years or more.

Interviewing

The interview aide-mémoire

An interview *aide-mémoire* was drawn up to guide the interviews, after initial discussion with disabled people and their partners during the pilot stage. The *aide-mémoire* was not intended to provide a rigid framework for the interviews. As the interviewing progressed some topics not originally included presented themselves and others, which were originally included, proved less important than it was thought they might be. Furthermore, it became obvious that there was little point pursuing some topics with particular respondents. For example, older couples whose children had been adult when the spouse became disabled rarely had much to say about the impact of this on the children. All topics were touched upon (where appropriate), but not all were explored in the same depth with all respondents.

The interviews started with a short, joint session with both partners. This covered basic socio-economic data – ages of the respondents, length of marriage, history of the disabling condition, numbers and ages of children, recent housing history, and the employment and incomes of both partners – which was used in its own right in the subsequent analysis. This session also helped the interviewers to get some 'feel' for the couple and their relationship.

The main *aide-mémoire* covered daily activities (including help with personal and physical care), informal networks, employment and income, the impact on and of children, personal reactions and feelings, the marriage and its current state, and service inputs and needs.

Carrying out the interviews

In order to explore the different experiences and perceptions of husbands and wives – of the disabled person and his/her carer – partners were interviewed first together and then separately. Previous studies of marriage (see Brannen and Collard 1982) have suggested that the best way to do this is to interview the partners individually, but at the same time. This process avoids either partner worrying about what the other is saying, or, partners 'collaborating' or standardizing their accounts. Couples were, therefore, visited by two interviewers – the researcher and another.

Wherever possible the interviewers alternated between carer/disabled person and male/female respondent in subsequent interviews so that, by the end of the fieldwork, each had interviewed roughly equal numbers of male/female, carer/disabled respondents. The two 'single' carers were interviewed by the main researcher alone.

Two sets of interviews presented some problems and were carried out in a different way from the others. One couple were first language Urdu speakers; an Urdu speaking interviewer was, therefore, recruited and trained in the use of the *aide-mémoire*. This couple, alone among those interviewed, were unhappy about the use of a tape recorder during the interviews. The interviewer thus made notes while working and produced an annotated version of the *aide-mémoire*. Consequently, the detail from these two interviews is not as rich as it was from the others.

In the second case when the interviewers arrived the disabled spouse (the wife) refused to allow separate interviews, despite the fact that this had been negotiated during previous telephone contacts with her. The data from this interview have been used only in conjunction with joint interview data from other couples.

Analysis

All the interviews, both joint and separate, were tape recorded. This generated an average of four to five hours of tapes per couple. These tapes were listened to by the main researcher twice; once immediately after the interviews in order that the data could inform the topics explored in the subsequent interviews, and a second time when analysis started.

The interviews were transcribed and the transcriptions checked against the tapes. Respondents' accounts were then assigned to a variety of analytical categories and transferred to index cards.

The broad framework was to some extent determined by the original interview outline; that is, respondents talked about certain issues because these were introduced by the interviewers. Other categories, by contrast, emerged directly from the respondents' own accounts; that is, they talked about things that were important to them, but which had not been initially addressed by the interviewer.

The framework of categories thus developed as analysis (and interviewing) progressed. Furthermore, as spouses and carers were interviewed separately, the framework for each was eventually somewhat different, although having a common core, by the end of the analysis.

The sequence of analysis started with experiences of respondents in the typical cases and then progressed outwards by steps, moving on to the next set of contrasting cases.

By doing this it was possible to address questions both about the commonality of experience of spouses and carers, and about differences related to their age, the spouse's condition, the suddenness of onset and duration, and the presence of dependent children. The analysis was, thus, continually testing out the uniqueness of any individual's experience against the possibility that that experience was common to other individuals in a similar situation or, indeed, to all respondents. Furthermore, by the end of the analysis it was possible to compare the experience of spouses against that of carers, and to examine whether *this* was affected by age, the nature of the spouse's condition and so on. In addition, it was possible to examine the role of gender as it interacted with these other variables.

Number of cases analysed

One case (one carer interview) was dropped from the analysis; this was the case referred to earlier where the husband had recently left the marital home. During the interview it was revealed that the spouse's condition was primarily psychiatric. The marriage was relatively recent (both partners had been married and divorced before) and the husband's mental health problems pre-dated the marriage by some years, although the carer appeared to have been totally unaware of this when she married him. The case was, therefore, excluded because it was so different from all the others and transgressed the original selection criteria.

In total the accounts of a total of 21 marriages (20 spouses and 20 carers, plus one carer alone) were included. In one other case (see above) the data generated were used only with other joint interview data. Consequently, the analysis is sometimes based on twenty-one couples, sometimes on twenty and, in relation to spouse's single interviews only, on nineteen. Where it is not obvious from the content, this is indicated in the text.

Characteristics of the couples

Age and sex of spouses and carers

Table A1 shows the ages of the spouses and carers by sex. This indicates that the sample tended towards the top end of the non-elderly age range. Although it is not strictly sensible to compare such a small group against population data, this age pattern is broadly similar to that revealed in the OPCS disability survey.

Because of the age differential between husbands and wives in the general population, the female carers were somewhat younger (average age 50 years) than their spouses (average age 54 years). The male carers were both younger than their female counterparts (average age 46 years) and nearer in age to their spouses (average age 45 years).

Table A1 Ages of disabled spouse and carer by sex

	M (n)	F (n)
Disabled spouse		
<34 years	0	3
35–44	3	1
45–54	3	1
55–64	7	3
Total	13	8
Carer spouse		
<34 years	2	2
35–44	2	2
45–54	2	3
55–64	2	6
Total	8	13

Duration of marriage

The majority of couples (16) had been married for 15 years or more. As would be expected, those who had been married for fewer than 15 years tended to be the youngest. However, there was one older couple (male carer aged 62 and female spouse aged 57) who had been married for only 6 years, both having been married previously, and one couple in their thirties (female carer aged 33 and male spouse aged 35) who had been married for 17 years.

Children

All but one of the couples had children. Given their ages, a surprisingly large number (12) still had children living with them. However, only seven couples had children at home who were still at school. The oldest offspring at home (29 years old) was a divorced son who had returned to his parents' home after his marriage broke up and had brought his young daughter with him. The rest of the independent children still at home ranged in age from 16 to 25 years. The thirteen dependent children ranged from 14 months to 16 years.

The spouses' condition

Table A2 shows the full range of the spouses' conditions or illnesses which led to their impairment. Some spouses had very complex sets of conditions and illnesses. For only nine of the twenty-one spouses was there an unequivocal, single diagnosis – such as multiple sclerosis, bronchial asthma or a prolapsed disc. Others had sustained injuries which had left them impaired in a number of ways, or had one condition which had later been overlaid by another, or had had some condition which had eventually led to another. For example, Mr Mead had an accident at work which injured both his back and his legs, Mr Hazleton had

Table A2   Condition/illness of spouse leading to impairment, by sex

Type of condition/illness mentioned	Number of disabled spouses*	
	M	F
Arthritis	3	4
Injured back	5	1
Chest condition	2	2
Arterial/vascular disease	2	2
Injury to joints/bones	2	0
Multiple sclerosis	1	1
Cardiac disease	2	0
Parkinson's disease	1	0
Mental health problem	0	1
Other	5	2
Number of spouses	13	8

* Sums to more than 13 and 8 because of multiple conditions/illnesses.

injured his back which eventually led to osteoarthritis, but became diabetic some years later, and both Mr Fowey and Mr Keighley had angina and later, possibly as a side-effect of the drugs used to control it, had developed colitis.

No spouse had a spinal cord or a head injury. Generally speaking the female spouses (who were somewhat younger than the male spouses) had different sorts of conditions from the male spouses. Four of the eight had some form of arthritis and all of these were (or had been) quite young at onset. This pattern is as would be expected given the epidemiology of arthritis.

The male spouses' conditions were more diverse, but included a significant subset (seven of the thirteen) who had sustained an injury while at work or whose condition was a known hazard of the type of work that they had done.

Because of the complexity of so many of the spouses' conditions it was often difficult to date onset with any precision. For example, Mr Alston had first injured his back 28 years before being interviewed and had left the heavy industry in which he worked soon after. However, he had found alternative work which suited him well and it was not until he sustained another injury, some 14 years after the first, that he left paid work entirely. Several men had continued to work for some years after their condition had first been diagnosed or they had first been injured, sometimes against the advice of their doctors. Furthermore, some spouses had one complaint for several years but had then started with another.

These complicated histories made it difficult for many spouses accurately to pinpoint any particular date at which they had become disabled. However, most were able to say that although they had had their condition or injury for *x* years, in fact it was *y* years 'since it started to get bad' or 'since it became as bad as it is now'. For the men this second point in time was often when they had finally given up work. Table A3 contains two sets of figures, one for original onset and one for the point which respondents identified as a significant stage in the development of their condition. This second column also includes those who reported a once and for all change.

Table A3 Duration of disability/illness

Years	Since first onset (n)	Since significant change (n)
>4	2	4
4–9	2	7
10–14	7	5
15–19	6	3
20–24	1	–
25+	3	2
Total (n)	21	21

Half the respondents had undergone significant change in the previous ten years although only a quarter reported original onset during the same period. Given this, it becomes more difficult to think about onset as being a necessarily meaningful notion when looking at the impact of impairment on respondents' lives. Moreover, it may be the case that onset proper has more significance for one partner than for the other. Mr Ibstock, for example, had suffered from multiple sclerosis for 15 years, but despite several major flare-ups of his condition during that time, for him, onset was four years previously when he realized he could not continue working. By contrast, Mrs Ibstock's account made it clear that the time when she discovered the diagnosis of her husband's illness had been both significant and difficult for her.

The majority of couples reported that the spouse's condition was deteriorating, albeit gradually (Table A4). To some extent it was as difficult for them to arrive at these assessments as it was to date onset. The condition of some spouses was deteriorating so slowly that it might appear stable, until compared with how things had been two, five or ten years previously. Similarly, a spouse with multiple sclerosis might experience very substantial fluctuations in condition over a long period but was, in the final analysis, becoming more impaired with each flare-up.

Table A4 Progress of spouse's condition

Progress	Number of spouses
Stable	2
Fluctuating	5
Gradually deteriorating	12
Rapidly deteriorating	2
Total (n)	21

The fluctuating conditions were mostly associated with arthritis and the two spouses whose condition was deteriorating rapidly had, respectively, multiple sclerosis and arterial disease.

References

Abrams, P. (1980). 'Social change, social networks and neighbourhood care', *Social Work Service*, 22 February, 12–23.

Allan, G. (1985). *Family Life: Domestic Roles and Social Organisation*. Oxford, Blackwell.

Anderson, R. and Bury, M. (1988). *Living with Chronic Illness: The Experience of Patients and their Families*. London, Unwin Hyman.

Arber, S. and Gilbert, N. (1989). 'Men: the forgotten carers', *Sociology*, 23(1), 111–18.

Arber, S., Gilbert, N. and Evandrou, M. (1988). 'Gender, household composition and receipt of domiciliary services by the elderly disabled', *Journal of Social Policy*, 17(2), 153–75.

Arber, S. and Ginn, J. (1991). *Gender and Later Life: A Sociological Analysis of Resources and Constraints*. London, Sage.

Astin, M., Lawton, D. and Hirst, M. (1991). *An Analysis of Pain in a Sample of Disabled Adults*. Social Policy Research Unit, Working Paper 825, 7/91. York, Social Policy Research Unit.

Atkin, K. and Rollings, J. (1992). *Informal Care and Black Communities: A Literature Review*. Social Policy Research Unit, Working Paper DHSS 778. York, Social Policy Research Unit.

Baldwin, S.M. (1985). *The Costs of Caring*. London, Routledge and Kegan Paul.

Baldwin, S.M. and Glendinning, C. (1983). 'Employment, women and their disabled children' in D. Groves and J. Finch (eds) *A Labour of Love: Women, Work and Caring*. London, Routledge and Kegan Paul.

Baldwin, S.M. and Twigg, J. (1991). 'Women and community care – reflections on a debate' in M. Maclean and D. Groves (eds) *Women's Issues in Social Policy*. London, Routledge.

Bayley, M. (1973). *Mental Handicap and Community Care*. London, Routledge and Kegan Paul.

Beardshaw, V. (1988). *Last on the List: Community Services for People with Physical Disabilities*. London, King's Fund Institute.

Blaxter, M. (1976). *The Meaning of Disability*. London, Heinemann.

Borsay, A. (1990). 'Disability and attitudes to family care in Britain: towards a sociological perspective', *Disability, Handicap and Society*, 5(2), 107–22.

Bradshaw, J. (1972). 'The taxonomy of social need' in G. McLachlan (ed.) *Problems and Progress in Medical Care*, 7th series, Nuffield Provincial Hospitals Trust. Oxford, Oxford University Press.

Bradshaw, J. (1980). *The Family Fund: An Initiative in Social Policy*. London, Routledge and Kegan Paul.

Bradshaw, J. and Lawton, D. (1976). 'Tracing the causes of stress in families with handicapped children', *British Journal of Social Work*, 8(2), 181–92.

Brannen, J. and Collard, J. (1982). *Marriages in Trouble: The Process of Seeking Help*. London, Tavistock.

Brannen, J. and Wilson, G. (eds) (1987). *Give and Take in Families: Studies in Resource Distribution*. London, Allen and Unwin.

Briggs, A. and Oliver, J. (1985). *Caring: Experiences of Looking after Disabled Relatives*. London, Routledge and Kegan Paul.

Brisenden, S. (1986). 'Independent living and the medical model of disability', *Disability, Handicap and Society*, 1(2), 173–8.

Brown, J. (1980). 'The Normansfield inquiry' in M. Brown and S. Baldwin (eds) *The Yearbook of Social Policy 1978*. London, Routledge and Kegan Paul.

Buck, F.M. and Hohmann, G.W. (1983). 'Parental disability and children's adjustment', *Annual Review of Rehabilitation*, 3, 203–41.

Bulmer, M. (1986). *Neighbours: The Work of Philip Abrams*. Cambridge, Cambridge University Press.

Bulmer, M. (1987). *The Social Basis of Community Care*. London, Allen and Unwin.

Burton, L. (1975). *The Family Life of Sick Children*. London, Routledge and Kegan Paul.

Clark, D. (ed.) (1991). *Marriage, Domestic Life and Social Change: Writings for Jacqueline Burgoyne (1944–88)*. London, Routledge.

Cooke, K. (1982). '1970 Birth Cohort – 10 year follow-up study: Interim Report'. University of York, Department of Social Policy and Social Work, Social Policy Research Unit, Working Paper DHSS 108. 6.82. KC.

Coughlan, A.K. and Humphrey, M. (1982). 'Presenile stroke: long-term outcome for patients and their families', *Rheumatology and Rehabilitation*, 21(2), 115–22.

Craft, A. and Craft, M. (1983). *Sex Education and Counselling for Mentally Handicapped People*. London, Costello.

Creek, G., Moore, M., Oliver, M., Salisbury, V., Silver, J. and Zarb, G. (not dated). *Personal and Social Implications of Spinal Cord Injury: A Retrospective Study*. London, Thames Polytechnic.

Croft, S. (1986). 'Women, caring and the recasting of need – a feminist reappraisal', *Critical Social Policy*, 6(1), 23–39.

Dalley, G. (1988). *Ideologies of Caring*. Basingstoke, Macmillan.

Dant, T. and Gearing, B. (1990). 'Keyworkers for elderly people in the community: case managers and care co-ordinators', *Journal of Social Policy*, 19(3), 331–60.

Davies, B. and Challis, D. (1986). *Matching Resources to Needs in Community Care*. Aldershot, Gower.

Department of Health and Social Security (Scottish Office/Welsh Office/Northern Ireland Office) (1981). *Growing Older*, Cmnd 8173. London, HMSO.

Department of Health (1989). *Caring for People: Community Care in the Next Decade and Beyond*, Cm 849. London, HMSO.

Dominian, J. (1985). 'Patterns of marital breakdown' in W. Dryden (ed.) *Marital Therapy in Britain, Vol. 1, Context and Therapeutic Approaches*. London, Harper and Row.

Duck, S. (1983). *Friends for Life: The Psychology of Close Relationships*. Brighton, Harvester Press.

Duck, S. (1986). *Human Relationships: An Introduction to Social Psychology*. London, Sage.

Dunn, P.A. (1990). 'The impact of the housing environment upon the ability of disabled people to live independently', *Disability, Handicap and Society*, 5(1), 37–52.

Edwards, F.C. and Warren, M.D. (1990). *Health Services for Adults with Physical Disabilities*. London, Royal College of Physicians of London.

Fiedler, B. (1988). *Living Options Lottery: Housing and Support Services for People with Severe Physical Disabilities 1986/88*. London, The Prince of Wales' Advisory Group on Disability.

Finch, J. (1984). 'Community care: developing non-sexist alternatives', *Critical Social Policy*, 9, 6–18.

Finch, J. (1989). *Family Obligations and Social Change*. Cambridge, Polity Press.

Finch, J. and Groves, D. (1980). 'Community care and the family: a case for equal opportunities', *Journal of Social Policy*, 9(4), 487–511.

Finch, J. and Groves, D. (eds) (1983). *A Labour of Love: Women, Work and Caring*. London, Routledge and Kegan Paul.

Finch, J. and Morgan, D. (1991). 'Marriage in the 1980s: a new sense of realism', in D. Clark (ed.) *Marriage, Domestic Life and Social Change: Writings for Jacqueline Burgoyne (1944–88)*. London, Routledge.

Finch, J. and Summerfield, P. (1991). 'Social reconstruction and the emergence of companionate marriage, 1945–59' in D. Clark (ed.) *Marriage, Domestic Life and Social Change: Writings for Jacqueline Burgoyne (1944–88)*. London, Routledge.

Gilligan, C. (1982). *In a Different Voice*. Cambridge, USA, Harvard University Press.

Glaser, B.G. and Strauss, A.L. (1967). *The Discovery of Grounded Theory*. Chicago, Aldine.

Glendinning, C. (1983). *Unshared Care*. London, Routledge and Kegan Paul.

Glendinning, C. (1985). *A Single Door*. London, George Allen and Unwin.

Glendinning, C. (1988). 'Dependency and interdependency: the incomes of informal carers and the impact of social security' in S. Baldwin, G. Parker and R. Walker (eds) *Social Security and Community Care*. Aldershot, Avebury.

Glendinning, C. (1992). *The Costs of Informal Care: Looking Inside the Household*. London, HMSO.

Goffman, E. (1968). *Asylums*. New York, Doubleday and Co.

Graham, H. (1983). 'Caring: a labour of love' in J. Finch and D. Groves (eds) *A Labour of Love: Women, Work and Caring*. London, Routledge and Kegan Paul.

Graham, H. (1991). 'The concept of caring in feminist research: the case of domestic service', *Sociology*, 25(1), 61–78.

Green, H. (1988). 'General Household Survey 1985: Informal Carers'. London, HMSO.

Griffiths, R. (1988). *Community Care: an Agenda for Action*. London, HMSO.

Grimshaw, R. (1991). 'From negative to positive: interpretations of children having a parent with complex disabilities', *Scottish Concern, Journal of National Children's Bureau's Scottish Group*, 19, 41–53.

Harris, A. (1971). *Handicapped and Impaired in Great Britain*. London, HMSO.

Hicks, C. (1988). *Who Cares: Looking After People at Home*. London, Virago.

Hoad, A.D., Oliver, M.J. and Silver, J.R. (1990). *The Experience of Spinal Cord Injury for Other Family Members: A Retrospective Study*. London, Thames Polytechnic.

Hunt, A. (1978). *The Elderly at Home*. OPCS Social Survey Division. London, HMSO.

Hyman, M. (1977). *The Extra Costs of Disabled Living*. London, DIG/ARC.

Jordan, B. (1990). *Value for Caring: Recognising Unpaid Carers*, King's Fund Project Paper No. 81. London, King Edward's Hospital Fund.

Kerr, S. (1983). *Making Ends Meet*, Occasional papers on social administration No. 69. London, Bedford Square Press/NCVO.

Kinsella, G. J. and Duffy, F. D. (1979). 'Psychosocial readjustment in the spouses of aphasic patients', *Scandinavian Journal of Rehabilitation Medicine*, 11, 129–32.

Knight, R. and Warren, M.D. (1978). *Physically Disabled People Living at Home: A Study of Numbers and Needs*. London, HMSO.

Korer, J. and Fitzsimmons, J. S. (1985). 'The effect of Huntington's chorea on family life', *British Journal of Social Work*, 15, 581–97.

Land, H. (1978). 'Who cares for the family', *Journal of Social Policy*, 7(3), 257–84.

Land, H. and Rose, H. (1985). 'Compulsory altruism for some or an altruistic society for all?' in P. Bean, J. Ferris and D. Whynes (eds) *In Defence of Welfare*. London, Tavistock Publications.

Leventon, S. and Jeffries, M. (1988). 'Children caring', *Carelink*, Winter, 3.

Levin, E., Sinclair, I. and Gorbach, P. (1983). *The Supporters of Confused Elderly People at Home: Extract from the Main Report*. London, National Institute for Social Work Research Unit.

Lewis, J. and Meredith, B. (1988). *Daughters Who Care: Daughters Caring for Mothers at Home*. London, Routledge and Kegan Paul.

Livingston, M.G., Brooks, D.N. and Bond, M.R. (1985a). 'Three months after severe head injury: psychiatric and social impact on relatives', *Journal of Neurology, Neurosurgery and Psychiatry*, 48, 870–5.

Livingston, M.G., Brooks, D.N. and Bond, M.R. (1985b). 'Patient outcome in the year following severe head injury and relatives' psychiatric and social functioning', *Journal of Neurology, Neurosurgery and Psychiatry*, 48, 876–81.

Locker, D. (1983). *Disability and Disadvantage: The Consequences of Chronic Illness*. London, Tavistock.

Lonsdale, S. (1990). *Women and Disability: The Experience of Physical Disability Among Women*. Basingstoke, Macmillan.

Mansfield, P. and Collard, J. (1988). *The Beginning of the Rest of Your Life: A Portrait of Newly-wed Marriage*. London, Macmillan.

Martin, J. and Roberts, C. (1984). *Women and Employment*. London, HMSO.

Martin, J. and White, A. (1988). *The Financial Circumstances of Disabled Adults Living in Private Households*. London, HMSO.

Martin, J., Meltzer, H. and Elliot, D. (1988). *The Prevalence of Disability Among Adults*. London, HMSO.

Martin, J., White, A. and Meltzer, H. (1989). *Disabled Adults: Services, Transport and Employment*. London, HMSO.

Matthews, A. and Truscott, P. (1990). *Disability, Household Income and Expenditure: A Follow up Survey of Disabled Adults in the Family Expenditure Survey*. London, HMSO.

McLaughlin, E. (1990). *Social Security and Community Care: The Case of the Invalid Care Allowance*, DSS Research Reports. London, HMSO.

Means, R. (1986). 'The development of social services for elderly people: historical perspectives' in C. Phillipson and A. Walker (eds) *Ageing and Social Policy: A Critical Assessment*. Aldershot, Gower.

Morgan, D. (1991). 'Ideologies of marriage and family life' in D. Clark (ed) *Marriage, Domestic Life and Social Change: Writings for Jacqueline Burgoyne (1944–88)*. London, Routledge.

Morris, J. (ed.) (1989). *Able Lives: Women's Experience of Paralysis*. London, The Women's Press.

Morris, J. (1991). *Pride Against Prejudice: Tranforming Attitudes to Disability*. London, The Women's Press.

Morris, L. (1987). 'The no-longer working class', *New Society*, 3 April, 16–19.

Morris, P. (1969). *Put Away*. London, Routledge and Kegan Paul.

Nichols, K.A. (1987). 'Chronic physical disorder in adults' in J. Orford (ed.) *Coping with Disorder in The Family*. Beckenham, Croom Helm.

Nissel, M. and Bonnerjea, L. (1982). *Family Care of the Handicapped Elderly: Who Pays?* London, Policy Studies Institute.

Oakley, A. (1974). *Housewife*. Harmondsworth, Penguin.

O'Higgins, M., Bradshaw, J. and Walker, R. (1988). 'Income distribution over the life cycle' in R. Walker and G. Parker (eds) *Money Matters: Income, Wealth and Financial Welfare*. London, Sage.

Oldman, C. (1991). *Paying for Care: Personal Sources of Funding Care*. York, Joseph Rowntree Foundation.

Oliver, J. (1983). 'The caring wife' in J. Finch and D. Groves (eds) *A Labour of Love: Women, Work and Caring*. London, Routledge and Kegan Paul.

Oliver, M. (1990). *The Politics of Disablement*. Basingstoke, Macmillan.

Orford, J. (ed.) (1987). *Coping with Disorder in the Family*. Beckenham, Croom Helm.

Pahl, J. (1980). 'Patterns of money management within marriage', *Journal of Social Policy*, 9(3) 313–35.

Pahl, J. (1988). 'Earning, sharing, spending: married couples and their money' in R. Walker and G. Parker (eds) *Money Matters: Income, Wealth and Financial Welfare*. London, Sage.

Pahl, J. (1989). *Money and Marriage*. Basingstoke, Macmillan.

Parker, G. (1985). *With Due Care and Attention: A Review of the Literature on Informal Care*, 1st edn. London, Family Policy Studies Centre.

Parker, G. (1990). *With Due Care and Attention: A Review of the Literature on Informal Care*, 2nd edn. London, Family Policy Studies Centre.

Parker, G. (1991). 'Whose care? Whose costs? Whose benefit? A critical review of research on case management and informal care', *Ageing and Society*, 10: 459–67.

Parker, G. and Hirst, M. (1987). 'Continuity and change in medical care for young adults with disabilities', *Journal of the Royal College of Physicians*, 21(2), 129–33.

Parker, G. and Lawton, D. (1992). *Different Types of Care, Different Types of Carers*. London, HMSO.

Pitkeathley, J. (1991). 'The carer's viewpoint' in G.Dalley (ed) *Disability and Social Policy*. London, PSI.

Qureshi, H. and Simons, K. (1987). 'Resources within families: caring for elderly people' in J. Brannen and G. Wilson (eds) *Give and Take in Families: Studies in Resource Distribution*. London, Allen and Unwin.

Qureshi, H. and Walker, A. (1989). *The Caring Relationship: Elderly People and Their Families*. London, Macmillan.

Richards, M.P.M. and Elliot, B.J. (1991). 'Sex and marriage in the 1960s and 1970s' in D. Clark (ed.) *Marriage, Domestic Life and Social Change: Writings for Jacqueline Burgoyne (1944–88)*. London, Routledge.

Rogers, C. (1973). *Becoming Partners: Marriage and its Alternatives*. London, Constable.

Rosenmayr, L. and Kockeis, E. (1963). 'Propositions for a sociological theory of ageing and the family', *International Social Science Journal*, 15, 410–26.

Sainsbury, S. (1970). *Registered as Disabled*, Occasional papers on social administration No. 35. London, Bell and Sons.

Sharpe, S. (1976). *Just Like a Girl*. Harmondsworth, Penguin.

Thompson, D.M. (1987). 'Calling all carers'. Survey, South Manchester 1985–6, Report (unpublished).

Thompson, P. with Lavery, M. and Curtice, J. (1990). *Short Changed by Disability*. London, The Disablement Income Group.

Townsend, P. (1962). *The Last Refuge*. London, Routledge and Kegan Paul.

Townsend, P. (1979). *Poverty in the United Kingdom*. Harmondsworth, Penguin Books.

Twigg, J. (1989). 'Models of caring: how do social care agencies conceptualize their relationship with informal carers?', *Journal of Social Policy*, 18(1), 53–66.

Ungerson, C. (1983). 'Women and caring: skills, tasks and taboos', in E. Gamarnikow, D. Morgan, J. Purvis and D. Taylorson (eds) *The Public and the Private*. London, Heinemann.

Ungerson, C. (1987). *Policy is Personal: Sex, Gender and Informal Care*. London, Tavistock.

Walker, A. (1982). 'The meaning and social division of community care', in A. Walker (ed.) *Community Care: The Family, the State and Social Policy*. Oxford, Basil Blackwell and Martin Robertson.

Walker, R. (ed.) (1985). *Applied Qualitative Research*. Aldershot, Gower.

Wenger, C. (1984). *The Supportive Network: Coping with Old Age*. London, George Allen and Unwin.

Wilkin, D. (1979). *Caring for the Mentally Handicapped Child*. London, Croom Helm.

Williams, F. (1989). *Social Policy: A Critical Introduction.* Cambridge, Polity Press.

Wilson, G. (1987). *Money in the Family: Financial Organisation and Women's Responsibility.* Aldershot, Avebury.

Wood, R. (1991). 'Care of disabled people' in G.Dalley (ed.) *Disability and Social Policy.* London, Policy Studies Institute.

Wright, F. (1983). 'Single carers: employment, housework and caring' in J. Finch and D. Groves (eds) *A Labour of Love: Women, Work and Caring.* London, Routledge and Kegan Paul.

Young, M. and Willmott, P. (1975). *The Symmetrical Family: A Study of Work and Leisure in the London Region.* Harmondsworth, Penguin.

Index